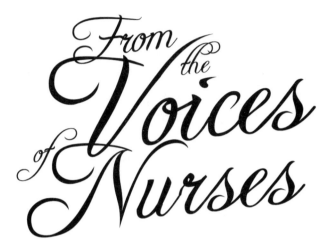

From the Voices of Nurses

AN ORAL HISTORY OF NEWFOUNDLAND NURSES WHO
GRADUATED PRIOR TO 1950

Marilyn Beaton & Jeanette Walsh

jesperson
publishing

2004

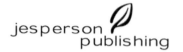

100 Water Street
P. O. Box 2188
St. John's, NL
A1C 6E6
www.jespersonpublishing.nf.net

National Library of Canada Cataloguing in Publication

Beaton, Marilyn, 1947-
From the voices of nurses : an oral history of Newfoundland nurses who graduated prior to
1950 / Marilyn Beaton, Jeanette Walsh.

ISBN 1-894377-10-9
1. Nursing--Newfoundland and Labrador--History. 2. Nurses--Newfoundland and Labrador--
Biography. 3. Newfoundland and Labrador--Biography. 4. Oral history. 5. Oral biography.
I. Walsh, Jeanette, 1944- II. Title.

RT6.N48B42 2004   610.73'09718   C2004-902463-9

Design/Layout: Freak Design   afreake@roadrunner.nf.net

Editor: Jocelyne Thomas

We dedicate this book to the 33 nurses who shared their stories and memories. Their
stories make us proud of their generation's contribution to nursing and health care in
Newfoundland and Labrador. They make us proud to be nurses.

Nurses quoted throughout this text are first referenced
by the year in which they graduated from nursing school. Complete
graduation information is provided at the back of the book.

Printed in Canada.

Table of Contents

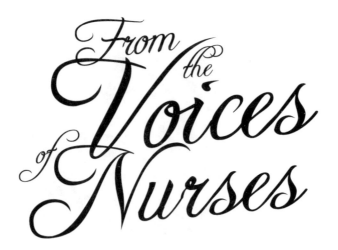

From the Voices of Nurses

AN ORAL HISTORY OF NEWFOUNDLAND NURSES
WHO GRADUATED PRIOR TO 1950

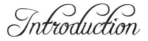

Introduction

Every project is motivated by some factor: in this case it was a chance encounter with one of the oldest graduates, at an annual dinner of our professional association. She was relating stories of her nursing experiences to a group of young nurses, and our immediate response was that other graduates of her generation likely had similar stories, and if not recorded, their stories would be lost to future generations of nurses.

Several nurses have written books about their personal experiences nursing in Newfoundland, but to our knowledge there is no documented record of the experiences of a group of nurses who practiced in various geographical and clinical areas throughout the province. Based on this assumption we decided to undertake a research project to record the experiences of these older nurses.

The focus of this book is not the findings of the research study. However for the purpose of the book it is sufficient to say that the research project received all the necessary ethical approvals. The research data will be published in nursing journals. The tapes of the participants' interviews will be stored at the Newfoundland and Memorial University Archives as a record of nursing in Newfoundland and Labrador and may be used as a source of data for future research purposes.

The intent of this book is to share some of the stories related by the nurses we interviewed. Their recollections/memories of events may not always be historically accurate, however, the stories reflect these nurses' situations and circumstances as they perceived them, and in that sense, reflect their reality.

To help in the selection of nurses for the project we defined the key parameter as nurses who had graduated from nursing no later than 1949 (the year Newfoundland entered Confederation with Canada) and who had practiced in the province. It was our contention that nursing in the province would be different before and after Confederation and that the recollections of these nurses would capture what nursing education and practice was like in Newfoundland as a country and as a province of Canada. Although all the provincial nursing schools and major health care facilities of that era were based in St. John's and many of the graduates tended to remain in St. John's to work after graduation, we endeavored to include participants who had practiced in as many areas of the province and practice settings as possible.

The interviews began in 2000. Potential participants were identified through the Alumni of the three provincial schools of nursing that existed prior to Confederation and the Association of Registered Nurses of Newfoundland and Labrador. Thirty-three nurses who graduated between 1924 and 1949 and ranged in age from mid 70s to 101 years were interviewed. Participants were included from all geographical regions of the province. Each participant was interviewed in their place of residence for one half to two hours, depending on the participant. There was a series of questions/cues to elicit information, such as "Why did you choose nursing as a career? What was it like as a student nurse? Tell us about your career in nursing." However, the majority of the nurses were very forthcoming with their memories/stories of nursing school, residence life, career in nursing, and often the questions/cues were not needed. Graduates from all provincial schools of nursing were included along with several nurses who had graduated from outside the province but met the criteria for inclusion in the study. Some of these graduates practiced nursing until the mid 1980s, giving almost a 60 year picture of what nursing was like in Newfoundland both as a country and as a province.

An analysis of the interviews revealed a wealth of information. As the themes of the interviews began to emerge, it was evident that we were not only learning about nursing and nursing education, but also gathering information about provincial social issues, historical events and life experiences that impacted the careers and lives of these women. Through their stories and memories these nurses revealed their strengths as women as well as their skills as nurses. The significance of the nurse in health care provision in Newfoundland became evident as often she was the only health care provider in the community/region.

What began as a research project into nurses' perspective of the history of nursing education and practice in the province became an enlightening experience into who our predecessors were as women and nurses, their contribution to health care delivery in the province and how the nursing profession had benefitted from their efforts. Despite hard work and long hours, their love for their work and their profession was evident in their stories and memories. While they were proud of who they were and what they had done, they were also very unassuming regarding their contribution both to health care and the profession, although several of the participants had received the Order of Canada and others had received the Queen's Medal, all in recognition of their contribution to nursing.

We acknowledge with gratitude the contribution these nurses have made to this book and to nursing in the province. While their stories provide a snapshot of the participants' careers, they also provide a glimpse into the nursing lives of hundreds of their colleagues from that era. From the perspective of the authors, and hopefully our readers, these nurses' stories will renew a sense of pride in what it means to be a nurse.

An interesting footnote to this book is that some of the most interesting stories were told after the tape recorder had been turned off. This generation of nurses had worked at a time when confidentiality regarding the patient, hospital activities and their colleagues had been instilled in them. Many were willing to share stories with the interviewer but were reluctant with having them put on tape or shared with a larger audience. The interviewers respected their feelings and agreed not to share any stories relayed in confidence, and in retrospect their absence in no way reduces the richness of this book's content.

PART 1:
Nursing Education

Any discussion of nursing education prior to 1949 must include the context in which the nursing schools operated. All three schools of nursing were located in St. John's and were hospital based. The oldest of the three was the General Hospital School of Nursing established in 1913. The school was affiliated with the General Hospital, which was sponsored by the Government of Newfoundland, and was the major referral center for the island. It primarily offered services to non-paying patients in all areas of health care except maternity, psychiatry and tuberculosis (Tb) care. The second oldest school of nursing, the Grace Hospital School of Nursing, initially offered an 18 month program in Maternity Nursing and established its three year diploma nursing program in 1929. The school, affiliated with the Salvation Army Grace Hospital, was operated by the Salvation Army. While considered a private agency, the Grace Hospital offered maternity services to non-paying patients as well as private. The third school of nursing, St. Clare's School of Nursing, was established in 1939. It was affiliated with St. Clare's Mercy Hospital which was owned and operated by the Sisters of Mercy. St Clare's Hospital offered general medical-surgical and maternity services primarily to paying patients. Only children were admitted as non-paying patients. Each school of nursing offered a three year diploma program, each with similar content and format. However, it became evident throughout the interviews that ownership and funding of the hospital influenced the students' education as nurses as well as determined other aspects of their lives as student nurses.

CHAPTER 1:
Choosing a Career

"I didn't like [leaving home] very much because I got very lonely and I didn't want to leave home... but I had to do something. So I came into training. I loved it!" Whiteway (34)

The interviews generally began with the question "Why did you choose nursing as a career?" This question elicited information not just about their career choice but also about the impact of their decision. The participants told stories about the preparations required to enter nursing, leaving home for the first time, and the costs associated with acquiring the essentials needed for nursing school.

Career Choice: As you will find with nursing students today, those who chose nursing in the 1920s, 30s and 40s did so for various reasons. A childhood wish, family tradition, fascination with the uniform were but some of the factors which motivated these women to enter the nursing profession. Nurse (44) knew as a child that nursing was what she wanted to do, "When I was 10 or 11, I really wanted to be a nurse and then as we went through school, the principal would say 'Are you sure you want to be a nurse?' But anyway...I really wanted to be a nurse. But then, by the time I got in, I wasn't quite sure. We used to have this little joke and we're going home Tuesday (laughter)! I don't know why Tuesday. But it was quite the shock, you know." For Moakler (45), it was the nurse's uniform, "You won't believe this but on Bell Island we had a company surgery...and I would see the nurse coming down over the steps each morning with her white uniform and her cape and her hat and I thought that looks some gorgeous. So I wanted to be a nurse." Both the uniform and family tradition influenced House's (47) decision to enter nursing, "My sister was 14 years older than me and she trained at the Royal Vic in Montreal. And I think it was her uniform at first (laughter). I was determined that I was going to wear a uniform like her...when I was about seven years old. And from then on, I wanted to be a nurse, you know."

During the 1930s and 40s, women who wanted a career did not have the choices that exist today. Women were expected to enter primarily female dominated professions, their choices were also restricted by family finances or geography. In many respects, nursing was an attractive career choice for a woman. Those who entered nursing did so as an apprentice, in that once the applicant entered the school of nursing she was provided for by the agency in return for her service. This form of education opened the door for many young women who might not otherwise have been able to pursue a career. Tobin (44), "I suppose at that time when I finished school, there were not too many choices available for us. Either you were going to be a teacher, a nurse, or you were going into the convent. So, I just decided that I would like to be a nurse." Bruce (43) also alluded to limited choice, "You did not have the choice back then, as you do now, not that it would have made any difference because I really enjoyed my training. My dad used to talk about nursing when I got into high school so it was sort of taken for granted that I was going to be a nurse." This external influence on the individual's decision to enter nursing was reported by other participants. When asked why she chose nursing, Sister Fabian (42) responded, "I think I was just asked if I would like nursing...the hospital was just opening and they wanted to find somebody who would be prepared for the future." In Godden's (38) case, her nursing career began as a result of the physician she worked with, "I worked at the Fever for years, not as a trained nurse...Dr. Milestone was the doctor and he gave me the opportunity to go to the General and train as a nurse and I did." Taylor (47) studied in England, "...right from the time I was a teenager I thought of being a missionary and I wanted to be a doctor...but that was during the war, the end of the war and women doctors were not too plenty and you couldn't get into training. I became a nurse. I didn't have any idea what I was going into."

For some, the desire to be a nurse was very strong and to that end they were prepared to do whatever necessary to fulfil their dream. Williams (35) pursued her dream to be a nurse despite her mother's misgivings: "I used to say, 'I'm going to be a nurse, mom. I'm going in for training.' And she said, 'That's what you're not! Go in there and the dirty old bedpan. You'd have to view all that and take it away from the patients.' She was... trying to turn me from it. I said, 'No mom, I don't think I'll mind that.' And she did everything in the world to keep me from going in. And I wrote a letter to Miss Fagner...she [mom] didn't know anything about it. I sent in an application and the next thing I got a letter back saying that I was accepted. And I showed it to her. 'Oh,' she said 'I suppose I'll have to consent to you going.' I said, 'Yes, I want to go in as a nurse'." For Mifflin (39) the desire to be a nurse was such that she gave up her teaching job to go into training, "I always wanted to be a nurse. I was a teacher for nine years. I wanted to be a nurse. I saved some money purposely so I could go. I really wanted to be a nurse and eventually, I am."

Whiteway (34) captured the mixed feelings that she and probably many of the respondents grappled with when making their career decision "[in the beginning] I didn't like it because I got very lonely. I didn't want to leave home...but I had to do something. So I came into training. I loved it." Regardless of why they chose nursing, each of these women saw nursing as an opportunity. While some responses suggest that the choice of nursing was not always an informed one, once undertaken these women pursued their career with commitment and pride.

Admission Process/Intakes: Having made the decision to enter nursing, admission to the school of nursing appeared to be comparatively easy. When one considers the rigorous process that students undergo to get into nursing school today, those interviewed revealed that the admission/application process was much simpler, although admission standards did exist. The common admission requirements to emerge from the interviews was that applicants had to be at least 18 years of age and had to have successfully completed high school (grade 11). House, "We had to apply and we had to be 18 and pass grade eleven." Several of the participants indicated that they had to complete an application and medical form, however, it seemed there was not too much structure to the admission process. In one case, the individual dropped in to see the director of nursing while visiting St. John's and was admitted to the program that day. French (39), "When I was a child, my parents never asked me what I wanted to do when I left school because they were always afraid I was going to do something and leave home. Anyway, one day I was in town with a relative of mine from Cupids and I told her that I was going into training. So, we traveled to the General and I asked to see Miss Taylor [superintendent of nurses]. When I went in and introduced myself and told her that I wanted to go into training she told me, 'okay.' So I went in and filled out my application after I was already in." King (48) shared a similar story when asked about her choice of nursing, a decision she made only weeks before the February class was to enter, "I worked in the bank [for six or seven months] and when I was interviewed, they did not think that it was going to be my life. I told Miss Oak that I was not happy at the bank and she said that

Jean Oak was going into training...so, I decided then to go with her. I had to rush and get all of my medical things done and I went up to the school, saw Miss Smith and I was accepted."

It was not until 1935 that students at the General School of Nursing were admitted to nursing as a group. Prior to that, students were admitted to nursing one by one throughout the year, usually when there was a bed available for them in residence. From 1935 onwards, there were usually two student intakes per year in September (B group) and February (A group). Depending on which participant you talked to, each group was either considered a distinct class or one class with two sections but most of the participants indicated whether they were in either the A or B class. In some cases, both groups shared lectures as they progressed through the program or where student numbers were really small. As a rule, both groups graduated together in the summer or fall of their graduation year. The number of students entering each class varied, with the larger group entering in the fall and a smaller number each spring. Class size increased during the 1940s, however, student attrition over the three years was high. Higgins (48) reported that 17 entered her class in February of 1945, but only seven graduated. Entry dates for a class varied each year with students entering as early as June for the fall class and January for the spring class. Bruce gives an example of some of the factors influencing the admission of students, "If I remember correctly, we were considered the first big class...there were 40 of us... there were two classes a year. One came in January and the other in September. The reason we did not get in until November was because I did not get my telegram stating that the entrance time was delayed. I believe it had to do with construction of what we referred to at that time as 'The New Home'."

Preparations for Nursing: Although the students' room and board were provided for once she was admitted to the school of nursing, getting ready to go in was the responsibility of the student and her family. Students were required to supply their own uniforms and other required items of wear which were made by the students' mother or purchased in bulk. Either way, preparing the necessities for nursing school was an expense for the family. Avery (45), "Now we were supplied with room and board and most of the clothing that we needed was bought in bulk before we went in. We bought uniforms, bibs and aprons in the package; we bought our stockings and underwear separate[ly]." When asked about preparations for nursing, Tobin responded, "My mother is a saint. We had to have four dresses which had to be 12 inches from the floor in your stocking feet. We had to have 14 bibs and aprons and then seven collars and cuffs that had to be snapped through the short sleeves at that time. My mother spent the entire summer measuring. We also needed so many pairs of flannel pyjamas, stripped pyjamas, slips and nylon stockings." Williams, "At that time, we had to get our dresses made. We were supposed to have two dresses, blue, and we were supposed to have four white aprons. My mother made every one of them...and she didn't mind one bit then. When she got all that done, she was so glad, you know."

Some of the respondents came into nursing either during or shortly after the Depression and the decision to enter nursing was not always an easy one for their family. Dalley (39), "When I told her I wanted to be a nurse mom said to me 'My dear, I got no money to buy you uniforms and stuff like that.' And I said 'Well, perhaps I won't have to buy them.' So anyway, one day I get this letter telling me all I had to get and the money it would cost. Mom said, 'Eleanor, my dear, we can't afford to give you that.' So I never said anything. Mom had a sister who was a teacher...and I said to mom 'I'm going up to Aunt Francine and I'm going to ask her if she'd loan me the money.' So that is what I did and she loaned me the money for my uniforms and stuff and to pay my way. She said 'Eleanor, if anything ever happens to you before you finish training, I'll never ask your mother for the money.' I said, 'alright Aunt Francine and my first cheque will come to you.' It's not that we were poor but there was a Depression."

Applicants were also responsible for books, shoes, personal items, such as toiletries, and once in the program, ongoing laundry costs related to the uniform such as getting collars and cuffs starched. Dalley, "All the laundry was done by the Chinaman...we had to pay for it ourselves. Some of it was expensive. It all depended on what you had done." When asked if she had to pay for books, Williams responded, "I had to have $50 to show when I got in training. My dad was a captain of a vessel for a man up in Harbour Buffet and, only for him, I wouldn't have been able to do it, my dear. Them times it [money] was hard to get."

Leaving Home: Making the decision to leave home to pursue a career could not have been easy. Most regions of Newfoundland were somewhat to very isolated prior to 1949. Travel was not easy. The nurses interviewed came from all geographical regions of the province as did the majority of those entering nursing during that time. Most of these women left home for the first time to travel alone on long journeys by boat and/or train. They arrived in St. John's not knowing anyone. When asked if it was difficult to leave home to go into nursing, Merrigan (39) said, "You did not know much, whatever you knew you were taught at home. I left one day in 1935...I can see mom now, up to the window crying." House was one of the fortunate ones, "I had never been out of Twillingate and then to go away into St. John's...I was lucky in a way because my mother kept a boarding house and a lot of people from St. John's would board with her. When they knew I was there they all more or less took pity on me. They'd take me out to dinner and take me to their homes."

Travel arrangements depended on the boat schedule, and in some cases, the individual had to leave home well in advance of the program's start date. This was the case for House, "We would go by boat all the way. Now, my class started in March and I had to...well it was frozen up in the winter and I left on the last trip of the motor vessel *Glenco* and went from Twillingate to St. John's, which was supposed to be about a ten-day trip. And then, I was in two months before training started, so they let me stay at the Residence and I worked over in the Admitting Office just to help out, you know, and I suppose to pay for my board. They didn't charge me board but they let me stay there until classes started." When asked how she got to St. John's from Woody Island, Williams responded, "We had to get in a boat and go to Swift Current. And there was a Mr. W.B. and he had...what I calls an old jalopy. I don't know if 'twas a truck or a car but there was only room for me to get up into it with him and that's who'd take me over to the train. The train used to come to Goobies and you'd get on the train and go to St. John's."

In some cases the individual might not return home until vacation the next year or until after she had graduated. This would depend on a variety of factors: the boat schedule, how much time the student had off, how far the individual lived outside St. John's, the weather and whether the individual and her family could afford the passage. While being away from family was difficult very often the homes of classmates in or near St. John's became a home away from home. Nurse, "And I could get home...and we'd all go home then. I remember I'd call my mother and say, 'We're coming up.' And she'd say, 'How many?' And I didn't know why she wanted to know how many. She'd have hot chocolate and the works for all of us to study. You know, I had no sisters but every one of them was just like sisters."

CHAPTER 2:

On Becoming a Nurse

"The nursing program was a far cry from the organized and in-depth academic programs today. But the problems of the past had to be treated with the same courage and the same tact as they are today…[the curriculum] was more than just lectures, they were making you an all round better person. You were marked on your deportment and passion." Sister Fabian (42)

Prior to 1949, Newfoundland schools of nursing offered a three year diploma program leading to graduation as a nurse. The program of study in each school was similar in format and content which evolved over time. Nurses who graduated in the 1930s received a somewhat different education than those graduating in the 1940s in that new content and clinical experiences were added. The nursing program was based on an apprenticeship model. Ward experience was a major component of the program and students worked in the hospital providing a variety of patient related services. Moakler, "I would say [it was] no longer than three months (before we went on the wards). It was work for service then, you know." The participants' stories clearly reflect the hospital's reliance on students to provide service and some might say that service took precedence over the education of the student. Yet, they were required to achieve a certain level of academic and clinical competency to graduate from the program. Whether or not the nursing program prepared them for what awaited them in practice was another matter.

Probation Period or Introduction to Nursing: Upon entering the school of nursing students began a probationary period when they were called a 'probie'(short for probationer). Some did not consider themselves a student nurse until they had successfully completed this period. The structure of the probationary period varied as did its length of three to six months. Those entering nursing in the 1930s were sent to the wards to work almost immediately with little or no preparation. Strong (36), "We did not have one bit of practical training at that time. I remember one month after I was on the ward I was asked to do the beds...I had never made a bed." Whiteway reported a similar experience, "We went right on the floor right from the street...the nurses showed you...we didn't practice or nothing...we just went in and did it (on the patient)." Although she also went on the ward immediately upon entering the school, Merrigan reported that ward duties were scheduled around lectures, "We used to do up the patients by washing them and giving them a bath...after we had our lectures. We would also give them their bedpans; we used to get a lot of complaints that the bedpans were cold so we would put some hot water over them to make it warm."

For those entering nursing school in the 1940s it seemed that the probation period was a combination of clinical and classroom work. As in the 1930s, students went to work in the hospital immediately, however duties assigned to the probationer did not require any formal training and could be performed by the 'probie' under supervision. Along with patient care, students performed duties which provided essential hospital services. This reflected a hospital environment where the nurse did all things (other than doctors' work) related to the care of the sick. Woodland (48) went into nursing on a Tuesday and "...on [the following] Monday I was on duty. I was only cleaning bedpans, changing diapers on the children's ward and feeding babies."

Avery provides a glimpse of the hospital duties assigned to a probationer in the 1940s: "We had classes every day. The first six months we did not go on to the floors. We were only permitted to look around. During the first little while that I was over in the hospital I was down in the central supply room folding bandages. We made our own dressings back then...we had to cut them...then they would make up the trays...and the things that came off the trays would come back to the central supply room and you would have to clean up the bowls and wash them. Finally, the trays would be made up and autoclaved. But we didn't get very much time over in the hospital [with patients] at that time. We spent most of our time in the classroom." Penney (45), who entered nursing school in August, gives some insight into how the students' education was 'fit' into the needs of the hospital, "The first day I went in, they sent me straight to the ward area...it wasn't a ward. Sister took me up to make sponges. In September, class started and...we had class every day, every afternoon, usually two hours...then we had assignments for the night, so we didn't get off duty until...well, you were fortunate if you got off at eight...you were supposed to be off at seven." There was little doubt that the probationers provided a vital service within hospitals.

Although classes were offered during the probationary period, their frequency and duration varied. Lectures and ward duty were so intertwined that classes were primarily scheduled during the workday in the students' time off and when they could be released from the wards. The probationary period ended with some form of examination and if successful, the student received her cap. Receiving the cap was a significant achievement for the student as it marked her first success in nursing and the cap was evidence of that success to staff and patients. Merrigan, "We had to work for the cap when we were in training...for six months. If you did not pass you were booted out." Woodland, "Well you had to pass all your exams...and then you became a student nurse. Before that you were a 'probie'." Successful completion of the probation period was clearly a milestone in the students' education; viewed almost as a right of passage.

Education Versus Service: Successful completion of the probationary period was an introduction to real life as a nurse; students immediately became part of the ward staff. As the school of nursing was not a separate entity from the hospital, a priority for the school was service to the agency and student nurses were considered a source of staffing. Ward duties came first and classes were 'fitted' around the needs of the ward or the students' work schedule. Following probation, students worked 12 hour shifts (often six shifts per week) on days or nights and usually had a two hour break. Even when working nights students were expected to get up for class and then go back on night duty. If the student did not understand the expectations when she entered the school of nursing she very quickly learned her role and adapted accordingly. Sister Fabian probably best reflects the students' acceptance of and adaptation to the responsibility, "In the 40s students did most of the nursing care even in their first and second years. I remember in training, we did take on a lot of responsibility. Looking back now, I didn't think I was taking on that much; I thought I was capable."

Expectations of the Student: The duties of the student nurse were clearly defined depending on the year or stage of the program. The color of the students' uniform identified the year the student was in and what duties she could be expected to perform. In the 1930s and 40s nurses did not have a myriad of medications to administer nor high tech equipment to monitor; their duties were reflective of the health care delivery of the day. For those who studied in the 1930s (before the discovery of antibi-otics) first year nursing duties focused on cleanliness with the goal of preventing infection. The importance of cleaning is evident in Whiteway's story of her first year: "You weren't allowed to do anything first...cleaning was the first thing you had to do. You had to clean the bathrooms. You had to wash the beds. We had to sweep the floors. We didn't have to serve the meals just bring around the plates. And to see that everybody had some-thing to eat (laughter). And there's a lot of things we had to do right. And you had to keep the linen tidy. And, if there was any mending to do, you had to take it to sewing room." In addition to nursing responsibilities, first year student nurses of the 1930s and 40s performed many tasks that today fall under the realm of support staff. Moakler tells of her duties as a first year student on evenings, "When we were on evenings...we had to make up lunches for the thirty patients, tea, and coffee and toast but the patients were marvelous in these days. I mean they'd come out and they'd help you to get the tea ready. Then you had to wash up all these dishes afterwards. Just wash them up, not sterilize them."

While the duties assigned to a first year student might not be considered difficult, it was the volume of work and scope of responsibility that could be considered overwhelming. On the job training was the teaching method used where students learned by 'doing.' At night students often worked alone with only a supervisor or graduate nurse to assist them if necessary. As compared to today, students were not oriented to their duties or ward routines but were expected to perform the necessary care for a ward of patients. Intensive care units and recovery rooms did not exist so students dealt with a broad range of acuity levels. The students were expected to work hard, adapt to whatever came their way and do so without question. Dewling (48) reveals what it was like for students immediately following the probation period, "The first six months we were helped along a bit, but after that we were thrown in the water and told to swim. It was kind of scary. My first night duty was on Alexander ward, which was pediatrics...from babies to 10 years old and there was 26 or 27 of them. I was alone and had never changed a diaper in my life so, someone showed me how to change a diaper. Also I did not know how to take down the side of the crib; I had no experience with cribs whatso-ever. After that there was nothing that would frighten me. After the first six months, we were on night duty alone...you'd get a report from the head nurse. Then, when she would say 'goodnight,' you were on your own for the rest of the night. I was never so scared in my life as I was that night. One of the things that I remember about that ward was not having enough diapers. We used cloth diapers and there was never enough during the night, so, about 4:00 or 5:00 o'clock in the morning, you were up in the utility room washing diapers and putting them on the radiator to dry so you could change babies again when they woke up. After a while I got used to that." Avery shares a similar experience, "It was scary first. I wasn't completely used to the Grace. Because the first months were in the class-room and then upstairs to the 3rd floor which was medical and I had been in the central supply room; but I had not had enough experience. It was like sending a baby away from her mother too soon. But I went out, and I did start to enjoy it."

Student responsibilities and workload increased in the second year although the general duties of a second year student's working days did not differ significantly from those of a first year. Additional nursing pro-cedures were introduced; the number of patients the student cared for increased and the students continued to attend classes. Both in the 1930s and 40s rest was key to recovery from an illness so many of the nurses' duties focused on the care and comfort of bed patients. Whiteway, "You advanced a little bit when you got to year two. You were allowed to do enemas. Of course, you weren't allowed to do it by yourself [at first]...patients were kept in bed for ten days and I would give four bed baths in the morning before I went to class." Puddister (47), "During sec-ond year we had a bit more responsibility, we were put in charge of eight patients who were all bed patients."

Although working alone on nights was not a new experience for a second year student, the increased workload provided additional pressure. Oakley (31), "Another girl and I were on night duty on the second floor with 42 patients. When they did the operations at that time, they had to come back to their beds and some were done late in the day and we would have them dying in their beds. I remember one patient in a private room was dying, there were only two of us on duty. So, we had to run back and forth just to see if she was still alive because that is all we could do." Penney also reveals the student's level of responsibility; "You were in charge of a whole floor as a student...we didn't have a graduate except the Sister who was on and she was in charge of the whole house. She'd be the only registered nurse we'd have on. You did the Case Room alone...all by yourself." Higgins related her experience on nights that nearly resulted in her leaving nursing, "I remember as a student it was very hectic, the 12 hours, and I know that one year…the second year, I did four months of lectures, two months and then I was off a month. I landed back again and that's where I almost gave up nursing. I was on the second floor of the old General and…there were 40 patients on that floor and there was a student assigned to assist me. Before the report was out, she was called down to outpatients and so I was alone with medications. You probably had two or three bloods going, IV's, and you had your medications at 6:30 or 7:00, your 10:00 o'clocks, lunches for everybody, back rubs for everybody (laughter). You were expected to do all that, and you were alone. You know, you had all that to do by 11:00 or 12:00 o'clock. The minister or priest always visited in the evening and you had to get a special tray ready and have that ready for the night supervisor to serve the clergy when he came but sometimes you were trying to answer lights and check on the patients and, in those days, besides what was going on routinely, you had all the Penicillins and shots so you had a tray of that to give, plus your medications, plus your IV's. So you had all of that to keep track of and to pour your meds for the next period." Mifflin aptly sums up the students' ability to adapt to situations such as these, "If you were on night duty, you would be on by yourself. But that too seemed second nature after a while."

The role of the senior or third student did not differ significantly from that of the graduate nurse; they could be in charge on days with the associated responsibilities. In each year of the program additional tasks were introduced with senior students being primarily responsible for sterilizing equipment and doing dressings. For some, third year was their first experience administering medications. Story (48), "[In] third year we were almost assistant to the head nurse. The third year student was the one who did all of the sterilizing and the scrubbing of equipment. It was quite ridiculous because here was a girl who knew everything and here she was scrubbing equipment. The night nurse's duty was to fill up the great big sterilizing machine and get it going so that when the third year student came on, she only had to put the equipment in." Bruce, "When we became senior students we would be in charge of the ward with supervision…if we wanted something or needed advice. We would fill out our reports, make sure the medications were given on time, and any patient that needed special care was looked after. Visiting hours was usually from 7:00 p.m. to 8:00 p.m., so, you would probably do a little bit of paper work. Patients were looked after for the night with back rubs and made comfortable and the lights were turned down. Then, at around daylight we would begin, what we called, tidying the ward. Fresh linens would be put out and whatever was necessary for when Sister came on in the morning to fill out her report. Nurse, "We had to boil in the big boiler the rubber tubing that was used for the IV's and make our trays up with forceps. So [as a] third year student really…it was the most work you did and the most responsibility of that was to have sterile trays. So you had to sterilize the big boiler and then you got the forceps and sterile towels and set up all the trays." In addition to her nursing duties, Tobin tells of other tasks required of a third year student on nights, "I remember when I was a third year student on nights we would have to go to the basement [in the dark] around 6:00 a.m. to stoke the furnace to make sure it was burning for the day staff. I used to be frightened to death! At night all we had to give out was an Emperin. The [medication] tray was only about six inches by four inches and we had all of the cards on that. The biggest thing you would have [to do] would be the dressings and stoops (a type of dressing)."

Scheduling of Classes: Classes were held throughout the three years and on occasion the A and B groups did classes together, particularly if the classes were small. Classes were usually held in the day, but not always, and 'fit' into the students' ward schedule regardless of where the class was held or where or when the student was working. There was little, if any, consideration of whether this might impact on the student. According to Griffen (47), "…you worked 'til 7:00 in the night…you might have two hours class during that time. And then, at night, you had to go to class if you didn't. We'd have probably an hour/an hour and a half class after supper. After 7:00 o'clock." When asked if she was tired in class after working 12 hours, "Oh, my dear! I'm tellin' you…I didn't know the difference. We didn't know what tired was, I suppose. It wasn't in our vocabulary (laughter)." When working nights students were required to attend classes. Students got off nights at 7:00 a.m. [with luck],went to bed, had to get up at lunch time, go to class in the afternoon, have supper, then be ready to report on duty at 7:00 p.m. for another 12 hour shift. Penney, "You had to get up in the afternoon to go to class. You just got up at whatever time class was; usually 2:00 o'clock. We had class and then we went to our supper and went straight on duty." Oakley, "We were on night duty and we would have to dress in uniform at 2:00 o'clock and go to a class. One day I had been on nights doing Ears, Eyes, Nose, and Throat. So, Dr. Carnell asked me to give the definition of yawning because I did a lot of it. I felt like throwing something at him." Classes were scheduled during the student's break period in the day so if a class was scheduled during those two hours the student did not get any time off. Woodland, "We got two hours off every work day…and [during] your two hours off, if you had a class, well it was tough. You know, you went to class in your two hours off." When students were out at other hospitals for clinical experience they returned to their home school for classes. Nurse, "There was classes every day and you had to get there from wherever." Classes at Memorial College were offered at night which meant the student had additional travel time. French, "I took chemistry [at the university]… and we had to be up there by 8:00 o'clock at night and we never got off of work until 7:00 o'clock. We had to be in at 10:00 o'clock and we had to walk up and down because we could not afford taxis. We would have our supper at about 5:30 p.m. or 6:00 p.m. and then we would go back to work until 7:00 p.m." Higgins also attended classes at Memorial College in the third year, "In the last six months before graduation students were like a senior nurse on the floor…you did everything with 12 hour duties and sometimes you went to Memorial for your lecture and you got back 4:00 o'clock and you really only had time to get ready if you were doing nights 7:00 o'clock. You had to get supper and go on at 6:30 p.m. so you were only getting four to five hours sleep that day, and this happened periodically during the week."

Class Content: The courses taught in nursing school in the 1930s and 40s were similar to those taught today. However, both the volume and complexity of these courses have changed dramatically for students currently studying nursing. The nursing program consisted of lectures and demonstrations by doctors and nurses in traditional areas such as medical and surgical nursing and obstetrics. Students were taught about diseases prevalent at the time such as Tuberculosis (Tb) nursing and in the absence of other categories of health care workers such as dieticians, students learned additional skills including the preparation of therapeutic diets. Each school offered similar courses with minor variations. For example, at St. Clare's students had a course called "Religion and Ethics," however these differences were more related to the philosophy of the agency than to the nursing program per se. Very rarely was theory taught concurrently with clinical experiences. Students might have classes in pediatrics or psychiatry long before they went to work in these areas and there would be few if any lectures when the student was in these areas. Those who graduated prior to the mid 1930s completed the entire nursing program in the parent agency although General students did go to the Grace Hospital for obstetrics but only when there was sufficient nursing staff to release them from the wards. Obstetrics would have been one of the few times when students had lectures specific to the clinical area in which they were working. Beginning in 1935, affiliations were introduced to the program where students worked in outside agencies to gain experience in services such as psychiatry and communicable diseases.

The curriculum was made up of courses such as Fundamentals of Nursing, Nursing Arts, Nursing History, Professional Adjustments, Medical and Surgical Nursing, Psychiatry, Pediatrics and Obstetrics. Science support courses included Anatomy and Physiology, Matera Medica (drugs and solutions), Microbiology, Psychology and Chemistry. Other support courses included First Aid and Emergency, Personal Hygiene and Ethics of Nursing. In addition to lectures, students had demonstrations of basic nursing procedures such as bathing, making beds, doing dressings and giving bedpans. Sister Fabian outlines the early curriculum for nursing students at St. Clare's, "There were formal classes...the major subjects had classes like Surgery, Medicine, Psychiatry, and Pediatrics. Some of the courses that we did included Personal Hygiene, Nursing Arts, Professional Adjustments, First Aid and Emergency, History of Nursing, Religion and Ethics, Microbiology, Psychology, Chemistry, Pharmacology, Doses and Solutions, and Diet Therapy. They were short courses of only 10 to 15 hours...that was in the 40s. We had 200 hours of Dermatology, Surgery and Operating Room (OR) Techniques, and Psychiatry." According to Sister Fabian, education in the 1930s and 40s had a broader purpose than just lectures, "[The curriculum] was more than just lectures, they were making you an all around better person. You were marked on your deportment and passion."

Given the emphasis on a university education for today's nurses, it was interesting to discover that nursing students in the 1940s did chemistry and dietetics at Memorial College where they were given lectures and demonstrations in these subjects. Dietetics was taught by Edna Baird and chemistry taught by a Mr. Hickman. As early as the mid 1930s, nursing students were taught dietetics by a dietician. Godden, "We had a dietician and we had diet classes...we went for Dietetics." However, it is unclear if she did the course at Memorial College.

The Teachers: Doctors played a key role in the education of nurses particularly in the early 1930s. In Oakley's case "...doctors taught my entire nursing course. I remember Dr. Burden's lectures. He said that Aspirin should be put on the poison list. We also had Dr. Bennett, Dr. Moores and Dr. Roberts." Whiteway was also taught by doctors but she recalled the role of the nurses in teaching students, "The nurse in charge of the ward taught us...like on the job training...there were no instructors then."

By the late 1930s, nurses became the primary instructors of student nurses although doctors continued to be involved in their education. Dalley, Mifflin and Merrigan, all graduates of the Grace, reported that "...the supervisors taught the classes...Miss Thomas, Miss Benson and Miss Strickland." When asked if she had been taught by doctors, Merrigan replied, "No. But one doctor used to give us classes over at Memorial. He taught us Chemistry." Ashbourne (42), "Elizabeth Bell Rogers taught Anatomy and Physiology, and Pauline Sheppard taught Orthopedic Nursing. Mona Smith taught Nursing and Genetics...Matera Medica. Classes covered such topics as personal hygiene, bedmaking, bathing and feeding patients. Mabel Smith was a nurse...she gave us lectures. She was more or less a teacher." Bruce, "Our nursing director did our lectures, and the associate director did a lot. We spent a lot of time in the demonstration room...learned all of our procedures." Avery, "We were taught by both [nurses and doctors]. Miss Vey was our instructor, she taught us nursing procedures and things like that. We would go down and go through all of the things that you would do in the hospital in your first year. We were taught to make beds, to dress babies, bath babies, do dressings, and give bedpans." According to Penney, "The Sisters [who were nurses] were mostly educators. I don't recall having anybody...a few doctors for classes but mainly the Sisters. We had a different Sister for each subject, and the doctors would come in. That would be in our second year we started having the doctors." Dewling, "There were several instructors...we probably had three. Pauline Sheppard was one of them...and there was another girl named Ford. Pauline did most of the clinical stuff and Ford did the principle and procedures. Doctors did the majority of our lectures as well as write our exams. Nurses had nothing to do with our teaching except for organizing it. Actually, nursing did not come in very much, except for how to do manual things. But we were good little mini doctors."

While doctors continued to be involved in nursing education, there seemed to be a clear distinction between what was taught by nurses and by doctors. The nurse teachers focused on the nursing content while the doctors taught the medical piece of the program. Each doctor gave lectures in his own speciality. Sister Fabian, "Doctors gave a lot of the lectures...they would lecture us for hours and that was a lot for the doctors to do." According to Story, "The doctors taught us mostly everything. The doctors did all of the teaching for free." Subsequently, the doctor's time became another factor to be considered when scheduling classes. Penney, "We would go out for classes sometimes because the three hospitals would combine. I remember doing psychiatry and having to go to the General for their lectures...because they used the one doctor...for the three classes. It was cheaper that way!" Woodland shares a similar story: "Then we went to the General for a few classes...Pediatrics and another one, I believe it might have been Public Health, because the doctors used to teach the classes. And it was easier for them to have them all in the one place. Dr. Tom Anderson taught Pediatrics, Dr. Miller taught Public Health."

Testing: Examinations were the method used to determine a students' knowledge and competency. Although students wrote exams throughout the program, two sets of exams seem to be particularly important: those written at the end of the probationary period leading to receipt of the cap and the registration exams at the completion of the nursing program. Students were tested using an oral exam or a demonstration of a procedure but mostly the exams consisted of written essay questions. Whiteway, "I was there six months before you'd get your cap. And you had to have your examinations then...in December and an oral exam and I had to put on a spiral bandage so I did it all and I passed it and I got my cap." Students wrote school exams which were prepared by doctors and often corrected by them as well. Nurses had very little to do with the examination of students and their work. French, "We just wrote the exams from the school and...doctors gave us lectures and we wrote exams on the lectures." Puddister, "We wrote tests and exams every term. Final exams were in June; the doctors would make up these exams." In addition to exams, Sister Fabian mentioned a report which was likely an evaluation of a students' performance on the ward: "Most of the lectures were given on the floor...the rotation was for two months. You had instruction as well as practical and at the end of your tour of duty, you were given an exam and then a report was written to the School of Nursing."

Registration exams were introduced in the province by the Government of Newfoundland in 1937. Even after 1937 nurses were not required to write the provincial Registered Nurse (RN) exams although many of the graduates did. Oakley did not have to write RN exams when she graduated and missed the opportunity to have them waived when the Association of Registered Nurses of Newfoundland was formed. However, in order to work she had to be registered so she wrote the RN exams when she returned to the province in 1956. "My girl was in training, so, I studied her lectures and wrote my RN the same time as she did." Oakley passed the exams despite having completed her program 24 years earlier. Whiteway also didn't have to write the RN exams when she graduated but opted to do so five years later: "There wasn't any registered nurses then [when I graduated]…we had a month's lectures before we wrote the RN exam. We had to write a paper…and we had to write on everything we didn't know anything about."

While the Government of Newfoundland administered the exams and licensed nurses, it was doctors who set and corrected the exams and signed the licensing certificate. Dewling, "I will show you my registration certificate; there is not a nurse's signature on it." Nurses had minimal involvement in the certification process of those planning to practice nursing in the province and subsequently, the registered nurses were very medically focused. Barron (49) reveals the medical orientation of the exams, "[The exams] were short and long answers. One of the questions was to explain about the procedure for artificial pneuomothorax…I knew it all anyway." Barron was diagnosed with Tb of the lung in her third year and had to leave the program for treatment. Her lung was artificially collapsed by 75% for two years. Towards the end of that time, she returned to complete her nursing program. During her two hours off each afternoon, she would take the bus (or hitch a ride) out to the Sanatorium, have her lung collapsed and be back on duty by 4:00 p.m.

In order to be eligible to write the RN exams, students had to complete a set of required courses with a set number of lecture hours in each course. Also they were required to complete a set number of clinical hours in their nursing program. Griffen, "I know when I went to write my RN I had been so sick that they didn't think I had enough hours. You had to have hours." Avery, "You had to make up sick time at the end. That is why I went home to study for my RN and then I came back to put in my few weeks that I had to put in." The students graduated before they wrote the RN exams which were written in November. This meant that students who graduated in August, September or even as early as February (and might be working outside the city), had to return to St. John's to write the exams. All graduates of the same year wrote together so examinations were held in a large hall, for example, Pitts Memorial Hall or Memorial College. The students wrote ten exams in subjects such as Anatomy and Physiology, Pediatrics, Orthopedics, Tb Nursing, Psychiatry, Materia Medica, Medical Nursing, Surgical Nursing and Obstetrical Nursing. By today's standards the examination schedule would be considered brutal. Woodland, "I know we had to write ten! We had to do one in the afternoon and one at night…five full days."

Results would not be released for some time after the students wrote. House,

"It would probably be two or three months before you would know if you passed." The results were announced on the radio and the names of the successful candidates were published in the paper. Those outside St. John's received their results in the mail. Passing the RN exams was clearly a significant event for these women. Whiteway, "They didn't tell us that we passed. You had to look in the paper (laughter). Everybody was waiting...then you saw your name in the paper (whew). That was something!" Woodland, "The whole class passed...I tell you how I found out. I was working on the children's ward and the grad on the first floor, who had graduated in '45 she came rushing in...and said 'The marks are out! The marks are out! I just heard it on VOCM! The RN marks were out. They didn't give any names.' And then Major Crowley came in and said she had a list of all of us. All the kids were jumping with glee" (laughter!) Once she passed the RN exams, the graduate then paid a small fee to the Department of Health and received a license to practice nursing. This practice continued until 1953 when the Provincial Government passed the responsibility for the examination and licensing of nurses over to the Newfoundland Graduate Nurses Association (now known as the Association of Registered Nurses of Newfoundland and Labrador, ARNNL).

Passing the RN exam opened the doors for those who wished to leave the province to work and there were many who did. Griffen relates the story of a classmate, "When Mary Bidgood went to the States, she didn't have to even write an RN down there. We had (whatever they called it down in the States)... she had enough credits from St.Clare's, to go right ahead into practice." Similarly, Higgins, "We did State Boards, you know... so that when we graduated, we had registration across with Nova Scotia and New York."

Graduation: Although graduation was a time to celebrate the culmination of their hard work, there was not always a lot of fanfare around the event. For those graduating prior to the 1940s, it was often a case of going to the office, picking up your diploma and pin and returning to duty. Prior to 1935, when nurses were admitted to the program when space became available, there was no fixed graduation date. An individual's graduation date would depend on the date she entered the school of nursing. Often it was determined by the hospital when an individual graduated and a nurse did not necessarily graduate three years from the date she entered. For example, if there was a staff shortage, the student's time could be extended until she could be released from the hospital. Strong was due to graduate in 1935 but because affiliations to other hospitals were introduced into the nursing program, she was required to stay an additional year to complete them.

Even in the early 1940s not all classes had a graduation ceremony. This was wartime and it seems that during this period some classes did and some classes did not have a graduation event. At the General, Ashbourne did not have a ceremony whereas Bruce did have one. "Before our class graduated in November of 1943, for some reason, they were not holding a ceremony. But for us, they set up a graduation course at Pitts Memorial Hall. It took place in the afternoon and we all wore corsages. We also had a graduation dance and a march where we marched in with our boyfriends. Someone asked me if I remembered singing at the graduation and I did not remember, but I did sing there."

Dalley, "We had a graduation…in Pitt's Memorial Hall. Miss Fagner was there…and a lot of the nurses. The superintendent of nurses on all the wards was there, and you could have so many from your family. But I didn't have anybody because my mother and father couldn't afford to come…I was the only one. Everybody else had somebody but me. Miss Fagner was sort of [an] administrator and everything all into one. They had lots of flowers…I had a bouquet there and they gave us a bouquet from the hospital." Griffen, "We had a very formal dance and a dinner at The Old Colony. We had a big graduation. I guess it was at Memorial or some hall anyhow…they had a little reception but then the next day, we had our dance. Before you met your date for the night, you had to be…the nuns had to see that your shoulders weren't bare or anything. They used to make sure that your shoulders or something weren't showing (laughter) because people had more…you know, drapes on them and stuff, telling them they were part of their dress, you know?" Woodland, "[We] had a graduation ceremony at Pitts Memorial Hall…and a dinner and everything. We didn't have a dance. My mom and dad were out, and my brothers…[from Grand Falls]. We graduated in July and I didn't finish training then until late September, early October."

Students were required to make up any time they may have missed before receiving their diploma which usually resulted in a delay in completing the program. Barron was told to come back from sick leave to participate in her class graduation ceremony where she won the gold medal for highest marks. She could not go to her graduation dance and it was another year or so before she was well enough to finish her program. Dewling, "I think they had a leprechaun down in the office to count every hour that you missed by being sick. Back then, you had to make up every hour to make the three years exactly. I remember, my finishing time was 2:00 o'clock on Easter Sunday."

CHAPTER 3:
Affiliations

"We went to the Fever Hospital…to the San…to the Mental. And we spent a month…and you lived there, moved bag and baggage…they were all nice."
Woodland (48)

Affiliations were a significant part of the diploma nursing programs in Newfoundland. The Oxford American Dictionary defines affiliation as a 'connection as a subordinate member or branch' however, in terms of the Newfoundland nursing education system, affiliations were 'an opportunity to gain clinical experience at another hospital in an area of nursing not available in their parent agency.' Affiliations to other hospitals were not originally part of the nursing curriculum. They became a required part of the nursing program at the General Hospital in 1935. There is no known documentation as to the rationale for this change nor what arrangements were made regarding the parameters of the experience or expectations of the students when affiliating. However, the General Hospital was Government sponsored and Government planned to open several cottage hospitals across the island in 1936. One possible reason for the introduction of affiliations was to prepare nurses to practice in these cottage hospitals.

The first affiliations included psychiatry at the Hospital for Mental and Nervous Diseases (The Waterford Hospital), tuberculosis nursing at the Sanatorium (the present site of the School for the Deaf) and communicable diseases at the Fever Hospital (near the present site of the DVA Veteran's Pavilion). Time spent in the operating room and pediatrics at the parent hospital was also considered an affiliation. Eventually affiliations became known as the opportunity for clinical experience in a field of nursing that required specialized skills. The duration of an affiliation varied from one to three months with an average of two months in most cases. Students were required to move to a residence located in or near these hospitals and live there for the duration of the affiliation.

Obstetrics was also classed as an affiliation, particularly by the General students. However, they did not live in residence but traveled back and forth from the General to the Grace. Obstetrics had been part of the nursing curriculum at the General since 1917 albeit only as lectures given by a doctor. In 1922, an attempt was made to have students go to the Grace for obstetrical experience but at best this occurred only periodically when the student could be spared from the General. Students were not guaranteed an obstetrical experience until 1935 when affiliations became a program requirement. All schools clearly viewed obstetrics differently from other affiliations. It was three months in length versus two and placed specific clinical expectations on the student. The rationale for this is unknown except that maternity care was a significant part of the nurses' role in the community and in cottage hospitals. A three month experience was probably considered necessary to prepare nurses wishing to work in these areas. Dewling's story supports this notion; "One of the things that we were supposed to do was to have 20 deliveries on our own without any doctor's assistance. We were supposed to be qualified to go out and be Public Health or District nurses. The Grace was very good about that, because if we were in the Case Room with a patient, they would let us stay around the clock and get all of our deliveries. We also did a post-natal course in the nursery. But for the Delivery Room, we were allowed to go in and out when we wanted to. The goal was to get them before you left the Grace. It was not all that difficult because doctors did not come in that much; most of the babies were delivered by the nurses, the doctor would show up on time to tell them [the mothers] the sex of the baby."

The focus of affiliations was not necessarily academic. There were token education activities and no formal lectures during the affiliation period. Generally, any classes the student received relevant to the subject were offered in the first six months of the program. There was little or no orientation to the agency and/or ward duties but the students were expected to take on onerous responsibilities. Higgins, "I mean, when I did my affiliation at the Grace...the first baby I delivered myself, solely, and the grad who was covering the floor...circulated and she had the responsibility of other floors as well. I remember the patient distinctly; she was pre-eclamptic and I had studied that but it was the first patient that I had actually experienced. So I spent the day with her and I remember that I had my notes and my textbook there and I was going over the pre-eclamptic patient...and everything went perfect. Because I had my lectures but I hadn't experienced the patient." Students learned 'on the job' from staff. Bruce, "There was not a teacher with us. We went on and the supervisor on the particular floor we were on supervised us." Dewling reported a similar situation, "No instructors came with us when we did our affiliation...we were at the mercy of the staff."

Although classes might not have been offered at the affiliating agency, students were expected to attend classes at their parent school. French, "When I went through training I spent three months at the Grace, two months at the Sanatorium...in the Operating Room and at the Waterford. That is nine months; the last year was when you did your affiliations. Also, we had two months at The Fever. I never did understand why we did not get our obstetrics lectures when we were affiliated at The Grace. When we took our psychiatric nursing, instead of giving us our lectures when we were in there...we had to get down the best way we could to the General. We would usually have to walk. We boarded at each place we went. But what I can not understand is why we did not get the special lectures when we were affiliated at the particular hospital we were at. I think it should have been arranged when we were there." It was the same for Roche (49), "I was at the Waterford for one month, the Sanatorium for one month, the Grace Hospital for three months doing obstetrics, and I was over at the Fever for one month. [We had classes] for three years. Even when we did our affiliations we had to go to class at the General." The same applied for students from the other schools. Penney, "You had to get there [to the General for class]...from St. Clare's. They didn't provide any transportation. You provided your own transportation. I think the General nurses were a little bit more fortunate. If they had to go to... the Waterford or something for lectures, and when we'd affiliate in the Waterford, we'd often get a ride out with the girls from the General because they had...well it was a truck...and we all sat in the back of it (laughter). Otherwise, you walked or got your own transportation, a bus or whatever."

For Oakley and Whiteway, affiliations were not part of their nursing program. Although Oakley had completed the midwifery program at the Salvation Army Maternity Hospital before entering their diploma nursing program in 1929. Strong was glad she was required to add an additional year to her nursing program to complete affiliations at the Grace, Fever, Sanatorium and Hospital for Mental and Nervous Diseases because the latter affiliation was the beginning of her lifelong career in mental health. Godden did not have to complete the affiliation at the Fever because she had worked there as an untrained nurse before entering nursing, "I didn't have to go to the Fever because I worked in the Fever for two or three years before I went into training." Not having to return there to affiliate suggests that the duties of the student nurse did not differ greatly from those of untrained personnel.

There is little doubt that the students were considered staff and provided service during their affiliations. From the participants' stories, it is also evident that there were differing expectations of students during affiliations depending on which school they attended. According to Sister Fabian, "...the affiliations would have started after graduation...the Sisters did not do the affiliations. But we did go there for lectures. It was a different age and we were not out in public so much but we did do lectures." Many of the respondents indicated that they completed the affiliations toward the end of second year or early in third year. This might explain why some students were given greater responsibilities than others, particularly if they were senior nurses. There were likely other differences in each of the nursing programs, but working and studying together during the affiliations gave students their first opportunity to make comparisons.

In telling their stories, the participants related experiences, provided information about the treatments of the day and shared their feelings. Tobin recalled various aspects of her affiliations which gives an idea of the students' experiences, "I can honestly say you did not get any information about the patient's history or why they are doing a certain procedure [at the Sanatorium]. [At the Grace] the supervisors did not give us much in the way of information. It was only observation. We had no classes. I really do not recall having anyone take us as a group and discuss a patient. We were the maids; we had to wash out all of the bloody linen after a delivery. We had our pediatric lectures before we went but that was the extent of it. That was the way it was for all of our affiliations...[information about psychiatry, obstetrics, pediatrics, and tuberculosis] was given...before we went out. That could have been given to you six months before you went to the particular affiliation. I don't ever remember getting a refresher course as a group when we got to our affiliations. The only thing that we had to do [at the Waterford] was a case history. Outside of that we did nothing to pass in. You took one patient and talked to him about his treatment, prognosis and medical history. The nursing assistants gave out the pills...the same at the Sanatorium; we did not give out the medications. I was frightened to death. I did two months at the Waterford, two months at the Sanatorium, three months at the Grace, and two months at the Fever... that was nine months in your third year." Nurse shares a similar story: "We didn't do any classes at the Grace, we just did service at the Grace...the Case Room, and I remember one thing...I loved the patients and I loved the nursery, you know, but we used to have to take the babies up in the elevator. I remember, we had to wash the blood out of all the linen at the end of our shift which meant sometimes, if you were supposed to get off at 7:00, you wouldn't get off 'til 8:00 or 9:00 (laughter)."

Woodland also provided a perspective of the students' responsibilities during affiliations, "We went to the Fever Hospital...to the San...to the Mental. And we spent a month. And you lived there; moved bag and baggage...they were all nice. I was scared in the Mental because we had to go up on the back wards with the medications. The students gave out all the medications and we'd fill a tray with the little glasses and the names and stick it in the little glasses. And you'd go up and you had to unlock a door and lock it behind you and they swore at you. And we had people who were isolated in cells by themselves and we had to go in there and give them their medication [nobody went with you]. We were really scared. [We gave] mostly phenobarbs and stuff like that...mostly it was tranquilizers, something to calm them down. But I used to be scared to death. At that time, we had classes in there [the Waterford]. And then when we went to the San, we had to do OR work because they used to do pneumothorax and stuff like that. And you'd really get to know the patients probably in a month. We had to go over to the old San and do night duty for the first time ever. We were the first crowd to give streptomycin. And the students had to give the strep. Maybe four or five...because there was a lot of us in there St. Clare's, General and the Grace. No problems with IM [intramuscular] experience there (laughter)!"

Penney reveals some of the situations that students could encounter, "We had affiliations at the Waterford...at the Fever...at the Sanatorium. We did three affiliations, two months each. That would happen usually between your second and your third year. [At the Waterford] it was more free...it didn't matter that you didn't have all the same discipline as you did in your school of nursing. [The people were] locked up...you went around to give the medications and you had keys galore and you unlocked the padded cells...I remember one time going in and the patient had pulled the padding out of the cell and she had a [lung] hemorrhage...she was an old tuberculosis patient. It was dreadful! She wasn't dead and she lived but, you know, how they bleed…and this was the warm smell of blood when we opened [the door]…and all the old padding which was straw and batten sort of stuff. And we didn't have a lot of staff. They had a lot of male staff on what they called the back wards but they needed them because they didn't have the medication and whatnot for those patients in those days."

Avery provides insight into the expectations of students, "Unlike most nurses in my class, there was nobody left to do an affiliation. They needed a nurse to go…to affiliate and I was only in my tenth month…it was the San, they were short. They knew that I had worked for 10 months in Cottage Hospital as a nursing assistant. To keep the affiliation open, they sent me. When they told me, for the first time, that I had to scrub for a pneumothorax, I thought it was brain surgery. But I did have somebody there to tell me what to do all of the time. It was a great experience."

Affiliations were not unique to Newfoundland nursing programs; they were also part of Hutching's (48) program in Montreal, "We didn't do tuberculosis although there was a San in Montreal at the same time. We went to the Children's Memorial Hospital for our pediatrics. When we went to the Children's, we stayed in the Residence there. And when we went to the Alexander down on Verdun, we stayed in the Residence there…that was the two affiliations that we had…we didn't see very many psychiatric patients in our own hospital at all. [You did obstetrics on the obstetrical floor] you had ten deliveries during your nursing training."

Of all the affiliations, many of the participants expressed feelings about only two. Generally they liked the San but the Waterford clearly evoked anxiety. House probably reflects the feelings of many of these young nurses; "I didn't like the Mental first. The first week I was there, every night we'd go off duty and I'd pull out my suitcase and…they'd say, 'Where are you going Pynn?' 'Back to the Grace! (laughter).' And they'd say, 'If you do that, you'll be sent home.' I said, 'I don't care. I'm not staying here!' I was scared."

Although the affiliations were often in environments unfamiliar to the students, their work did not necessarily differ from that in the parent hospital. They were given onerous responsibilities but assumed them without question and performed them to the best of their abilities. As with the other challenges they faced throughout their nursing program, the students demonstrated their resilience and ability to adapt regardless of what they encountered.

CHAPTER 4:

Life as a Student

"I lived in residence, we became very attached to each other. We depended on each other to talk about all our problems." Avery (45)

While the nursing education programs in the province were generally the same in structure and content, life as a nursing student varied depending on which school the student attended. The Grace and St. Clare's Hospitals were both privately operated and did not have access to the same resources as the General Hospital which was Government sponsored. Access to resources was evident in the benefits students received during their three years of nursing school as well as how they impacted on the students' work and social life. Differences became evident when students began to share clinical experiences such as affiliations and and from them make comparisons. However, the respondents' stories suggest these differences only added to the student experience.

When these young women made the decision to choose nursing as a career, it was not just about getting an education it was taking on a way of life. While nursing had a lot to offer them, things did not come easily. As apprentices, they worked long hours, got paid very little (if any money) and really were at the mercy of those in charge. And yet as they had adapted to the duties and responsibilities in the hospital, so did they adapt to life as a student. They made the most of what they had in terms of time off and money to spend and created memories that are as vivid for them today as the day they happened. Most importantly, these women established a circle of life long friends. Despite the hard work, they had fun, albeit 'innocent fun' (as they called it) and came up with creative ways of 'adapting to the system.'

Life in Residence: Living in residence was as much a part of the student experience as the classroom and clinical piece. Students were required to live in residence even if they lived near the school. The only time they could return home to stay was during vacation. Residence accommodations varied from living in a nurses' residence to living in houses near the hospital. Sister Fabian states that at St. Clare's "[...all the nurses lived in residence]. We did not have a residence, as such, at that time; we had dwelling homes. One was on LeMarchant Road and the larger one was on St. Clare Avenue." Oakley lived in "...one big room where all of us slept. All of our nurses stayed in the big dormitory." As the class size increased, students from the Grace lived in residence for a while but then moved to houses near the hospital. According to Merrigan, "We lived outside in a house [when they did not have room in residence]. They [the hospital] paid the rent." Dalley shares a similar story "I stayed in residence there...they didn't really have a residence then. At that time they started one. We stayed in a house across the street called 'Vasto's Place' or something. We didn't have to pay for it...we'd eat over there...before I finished they had the residence built." House, "The first six months, we were in the dorm; there was eight of us. Then, after that, we moved out probably two in a room or four in a room (laughter)."

Students at the General also lived in a residence for nurses. Graduate nurses also lived there but in a separate wing from the other students. Whiteway, "Well, first you went into the dungeon, you'd say...with four beds. But after a while you'd get your own room. That's when you moved up [from year to year]." It was the practice for all the schools to have nurses working nights separated. King lived in the "...Merchant Navy residence when doing nights. We liked it there because we were away from the hospital. [We] did three months night duty [and] rarely had a chance to sleep in." Sister Fabian, "The night nurses stayed on Patrick Street. They would move residence when they were on nights. But that only happened for a couple of years." Woodland, "We had a great esprit de corps. I enjoyed residence life. I didn't for the first few months because, you know, you're home sick and everything else but, once I got settled down...my three years just seemed to fly by. You had three and four in a room. And when you went in first, you had a dorm. It was about seven or eight beds in it. And then you graduated to three bedrooms and four bedrooms (laughter). Well, you also had night-duty rooms, as we used to call them. They were up on the third floor, and when you went on night duty, you had to move up to these rooms...less noise. But we had to do night duty so often that they cut that out (laughter). You had to stay in your own room!"

Living in residence had a different meaning for each of these women. For those from rural Newfoundland it was a home away from home; for some it was a place to share with their 'other' family, while for others it was a place to sleep. For the majority, living in residence was a positive experience. Penney, "[We] lived in residence...that was nice. I enjoyed...it was great discipline, of course (laughter)." Avery, "I lived in residence. We became very attached to each other. We depended on each other to talk about all of our problems." Those who lived in or had family in St. John's had other options. Whiteway, "I lived in residence but I had my grandmother and my aunts who all lived together in St. John's. So when I'd get off, I'd head straight for home (laughter). We [the students] used to go out together. We were very close." Story, "I slept there [in residence] but I did not spend much time there. I was home and out every minute I could be. I was not one for hanging around in the residence. We [the students] would go over the hill and take a walk." Nurse, "[Residence] was quite involved because we were one big family because we were a small class; there was only twelve of us. You weren't allowed to go home, not for overnight. I used to go home in two...a couple of hours off....go home and wash my hair and find myself running home...or a fast trot...because I lived on the corner of Prescott and the hospital was fifteen minutes fast-walk away. Higgins, "[Residence life] was wonderful....we used to have...great times together."

Like the nursing program, residence life was very structured and often the rules didn't make a whole lot of sense but students quickly learned to adapt. When on nights, they were expected to sleep so many hours and could not get up until the designated time. Whiteway, "And you had to go to bed every morning after breakfast and you weren't allowed to get up until 2:30 p.m. whether you were awake or not. There was always somebody checking on you." Penney, "...and then you had to get up, of course, in the afternoon to go to class. But you weren't allowed to go out, of course, before that time (laughing). You got up whatever time class was, usually 2:00 o'clock."

Nightly curfew in all the schools was 10:00 p.m. and students had to be in bed no later than 10:30 p.m. House, "[They] were strict. We had to be in at 10:00 o'clock at night and, of course, there was no males whatever allowed in the residence at the Grace...and 10:00 o'clock we had to be in our rooms." Penney, "We had to be in, of course, at quarter to 10:00 p.m. They said 10:00 o'clock but, I mean, quarter to 10:00 p.m. you were really expected because you had to be in bed by...Sister Brown said 10:00 p.m. and...lights were out. So then you usually got up in the store loft and got into the clothes cupboard and turned on the light to do a bit of studying (laughter). But...you were in bed. It was a healthy life I suppose...you couldn't do much in the way of socializing because, as I say, you didn't get off duty. You were supposed to get off at 7:00 a.m. and it was very infrequently you'd get off at 7:00 a.m." Moakler, "We had to be in bed because...the housemother would make rounds. So you had to be in bed, we stayed in bed most of the time (laughter). But I lived on Bell Island and my parents were very good to me. They would send me a parcel every Thursday and in the parcel would be a roast of beef or a roast of pork or a chicken and different other things...because we were always hungry in training. And I remember one time it didn't arrive on Thursday. It arrived on Friday. And, in these days, Catholics didn't eat meat on Friday, so nobody could have it because everybody would have some of it. We went to bed that night and about 12:00 o'clock we could hear all the clocks alarming...and everybody piled in the room to get the parcel out for a bit of food. We had a lot of fun....a lot of innocent fun." Packages from home were always welcome and shared. Merrigan, "...but what you got from your parents would help. Sometimes they would send chicken or something like that. Most of the girls had somebody sending them stuff."

Time Off: When asked about time off, the respondents viewed any time away from the wards as time off including the break during their shift, time off during the week, and vacation time. They also discussed the factors which affected their time off such as curfews and late leaves. Individual recollections of time off varied but collectively the stories give a sense of how much free time the students actually got. Students worked 12 hours shifts usually with a two hour break in the morning or afternoon. This was considered time off even though they were usually required to attend class. If they worked nights, there was also a break but not if someone was off sick. For nursing students in the 1930s, time off was rare. Whiteway reported that "...first when I went there, you used to work all day from 7:00 a.m. to 7:00 p.m...and six days. We'd get one day off every two weeks. And you got three hours off on Sunday to go to church. And every second Sunday off." Dalley tells a similar story; "We'd have no days off. We'd just have these two hour breaks. We'd work seven days a week."

The majority of respondents who graduated in the 1940s reported that they got a half day off each week and a full day off every other week, which was usually Sunday. Penney describes the half day off, "We got what they called a 'PM' and it started at 2:00 o'clock...that was what you got off...from 2:00 p.m. to 7:00 p.m. I suppose, you know, we were young and had lots of energy and it never seemed we got tired although, now as I look back on it, (laughter) I wonder, you know?" Woodland, "Sometimes you'd get a 4:30 p.m. off which was real good (laughter). That would be only occasionally. And a half-day a week starting at 1:00 o'clock...every week. When we went in on Monday it was posted and you'd know that you had Thursday afternoon off or Tuesday afternoon." The students' day off was limited by the nightly curfew although they were permitted an occasional late leave. Time off was not always consistent and varied between the schools. Griffin, "And you got a half day off a week, if you were lucky. That was it...and then your late leave you had to be in bed by 9:00 p.m. but, on late leave which you got...during the summer because you didn't have class, you got it for 10:30 p.m." Tobin, "We had to be in at 10:00 p.m. except on Friday and Saturday, we were allowed out until 10:30 p.m. We were allowed one late leave per month, which was until 12:00 a.m." Once they entered nursing students were only permitted to sleep at home during vacation. There were no overnights or weekends off even for students who lived in or near St. John's. House, "We had half day [off] a week. We would never get an overnight or a weekend." Higgins, "...and even when you had your day off or afternoon off or whatever, you had to be in at 10:00 o'clock. We got one half day per week, no overnights or weekends to go home and...the only time you slept home was when you had your two or three weeks holidays, so for the whole year, for three years, you...lived in residence with only your vacation time." Nurse, "...and you got one late leave a month...until 12:00 a.m., no overnight. There was no such thing, even though I lived in St. John's."

As the students were a primary source for staffing, vacation depended on whether there was sufficient staff to relieve a student for an extended period of time. Where and how the student spent her vacation depended on the distance a student had to travel to get home, how much time she had off and whether she could afford the transportation costs. Students got vacation after they were in the program for one year. The length varied from two weeks to a month with an average of three weeks. Students from rural Newfoundland usually got their vacation in the summer, particularly if they were dependent on the boats for transportation. Although there were those who did not go home for vacation for the three years they were in nursing school. According to Tobin, "Vacations were scheduled around the availability of transportation. Those who had to travel by boat would have their vacation planned according to the boat schedule...which was often erratic. Those living in town usually would have vacation scheduled around Christmas...three weeks." Dalley, "We'd get our summer holidays, [for] two weeks I would go to Moreton's Harbor. They'd come up to Lewisporte in a boat after me...the train would only come to Lewisporte." Penney, "We got...really no vacation. I got vacation the middle year I was in. We didn't get any the first year I was there and the second year, we got two weeks and the last year, because you were graduating, we just didn't get any. Two weeks in three years, yeah."

Stipend: In keeping with an apprenticeship model, students received a stipend which varied in amount depending on which year the student was in and which school the student attended. Ability to pay students a stipend depended on availability of resources so it is not surprising that students in privately operated schools did not always fare as well as those in the government sponsored agency. Students were housed and fed at no cost and this comprised a portion of their stipend. Specifics about the amount of the stipend varied, however, it was obvious that the stipend in no way reimbursed the students' long hours and hard work. Oakley, "I did [get paid] because I was an officer but the rest did not get paid. [Yes] they did...get something. I remember that now." Williams who also trained at the Grace indicated that they did not get paid until third year: "Never got anything! I think the last year I was there in training, I got $8.00 a month." Whiteway, "You got $3.50 I think the first year and $8.00 the second year and $13.00 in third year." Those women who graduated in late 1930s and early 1940s received more money. Mifflen, "When you went into nursing school, you worked the first six months for nothing. After six months you got $11.00 a month or something, just enough to keep you in pocket money. Our board did not cost us anything. But that is all we used to get was the $11.00 a month pocket money until we finished." Penney, "[We did not get paid] not one cent. We got $1.00 with our Christmas card at Christmas...I remember that. The other hospitals did get some remuneration but we didn't...you were frugal...you watched your money (laughing)." Avery, "While I was in training, we were as poor as church mice, but the first two years we got $5.00 a month and the last year we got $7.00 a month. Now we were supplied with room and board...things were not so expensive then; you could get more for your dollar. We found that we could buy a package of cigarettes here and there and almost everyone in residence would own them." Woodland, "We got $5.00 a month (laughter)! And then it went up to $12.00 and then it went up to $16.00...it was a bit of pocket money." King, "As a student we were paid $12.00 a month in first year, then it went up to $15.00 in second year and about $18.00

in the third year."

In the privately operated schools, students had to be careful or they would find that they spent their stipend for reasons other than entertainment. Woodland, "I don't know about the other hospitals...if we broke thermometers or syringes or something, we had to replace them. And one time, I broke a 50 cc syringe and oh...I had to pay for it. [It would cost]...more money than I ever had (laughter)! So I went over to the drugstore to Mr. Janes, a lovely man was right across the street. And I said 'I broke a 50 cc syringe and I got to pay x number of dollars for it.' He said 'What nonsense!' And he gave it to me for $10.00. So I took the syringe back and replaced it (laughter)! That was two months' salary." Griffen tells a similar story; "I remember the day I had enough sick time in, I was finished, and...I was in the OR and dropped the thing of syringes and, at that time, I mean, you spent more time on Water Street looking for cups and saucers that you broke. You had to replace everything you broke. Spend your only money and you had none. We got $1.00 Christmas (laughter)...every Christmas. I had $3.00 while I was in there... but this day I dropped the thing of syringes. I remember Dr. Murphy saying, 'Oh my, I wouldn't like to be in your shoes now.' So I went over after I was finished work...to get my pin...I remember Sister saying, 'Mm! You're finishing now, and just look how much money you owe us because of breaking those syringes today.' And, of course, I was always saucy I suppose, so I said, 'Now, that's nothing to what it cost my father.' So she gave me my things...(laughter). She didn't charge me for them after all. She could be still billing me, I suppose (laughter). But I had no intention of paying for those syringes. If you broke anything, you had to replace it or pay for it."

Social Life: Despite limited money, long work hours and very little freedom, students made the most of their free time; they made every minute count. Their stories tell of a more innocent time when you created your own fun and made the most of what you had in the way of resources. The stories tell of the role of the house mother in the life of the student and the control the school had over the students' off time, their dress and with whom they socialized. Oakley, "We did not mind it [the hard work]. Half of the time we would have a lot of outport patients who did not have any family in St. John's. I used to spend hours in the laundry washing out their pajamas...when we would go off in the evenings. But of course, they had nobody else to do it, I suppose. Every Saturday I used to get $5.00 a week and we would walk down Water Street and go into every store. Then we would come up to the restaurant that was up by the post office where we would spend 50 cents. We had a wonderful time." Dalley, "The most I did [in that two hours] was rest. If you wanted anything at the store, we'd go as far as the store...usually go down to the Chinaman's and get our cuffs and collars. Avery, "We went to the Cosmopolitan for cake and a drink. It was a place with booths where you could eat. It was about four doors down Pleasant Street on the side of the Grace. We could go down there and have our smoke if we wanted to. I learned to smoke at that place. Cigarettes were not that expensive; we could have a drink in our two hours off. We would not buy anything big; you could get a pair of stockings. You would not be able to walk through the door with $5.00 today." King, "There was not a great deal to do. We would get off at 7:00 p.m. and get out of there around 7:30 p.m. We would walk up by Rawlins Cross and there was an ice cream place there called, 'Diana Sweets' where we would have our ice cream sodas. Then, we would run down Military Road and Forest Drive and get in by 10:00 p.m." Woodland, "You'd try to get the same afternoon off that your friend had off so you could go to a movie and out to have a bite to eat or something."

Other Influences: The profession of nursing evolved from both a military perspective, i.e. Florence Nightingale and the Crimean War, and a religious perspective, i.e. the hospices established by religious orders in the middle ages. Schools of nursing in Newfoundland were founded on both perspectives; the General Hospital with its military connection and both the Grace and St. Clare's evolving from their religious, missionary philosophies. Needless to say, both perspectives had significant influence on the students' education and their formation as young women. Prayers or Mass played a major role in the daily life of students attending the two latter schools. At the General, while church attendance was a part of the students' life, usually it was a weekly activity on Sunday when students would be given time off to attend church. Oakley, "We were called at 6:00 a.m. and went to prayers and breakfast. We were on the floor for 7:00 a.m." Dalley, "Every morning we'd have to go down to the auditorium for prayers. If we were a few minutes late, we didn't mind...but if Miss Fagner was having prayers...we'd try to find out every night before we'd go to bed...who was having prayers in the morning. And this morning...I knew Miss Fagner was going to have prayers and I got up and got ready...and I was downstairs. All our nurses were down there waiting for her to come because nobody would be late 'cause...for sure you were going to lose your free time. By and by in she walks. She looked up and she said 'Miss Jennings, you'll lose your free time today.' And everyone of the nurses looked and couldn't figure out what it was about and I didn't either. She said, 'Go up and get your cap.' I didn't have my cap on! And everyone of the nurses were all there and not one of us noticed it! And I lost two hours." Moakler, "If you worked with Mary Feehan, you wouldn't get a half day during the week because you had to go to church on Sunday mornings because Mary Feehan made sure that, being a Catholic girl, you had to go down to St. Joseph's. [You always got] ...Sunday mornings."

In keeping with the military influence, the students' day began with roll call and inspection each morning before going on duty. Barrett (41), "I mean under Miss Rogers, we had to wear hairnets. And your hair had to be up. And, if it was down, you were sent off duty. And you were inspected. And your rooms were inspected." Penney, "We worked from 7:00 a.m. to 7:00 p.m. and we were up at 6:00 a.m...roll call was 6:00 a.m. We went over for roll call and Sister checked us to see that we had our [hair] nets on and our apron was on properly and the right length...every morning. We had inspection first, at 6:00 a.m., and then we went down to Mass and then we'd come up and have our breakfast and went on duty." Woodland, "We had prayers at 6:300 a.m. Roll call, prayers [every morning]...and if you missed (laughter) you lost your late leave! [That was]...11:45 a.m...once a week."

The most pronounced military influence was the distinction between students and staff; what could be referred to as the pecking order. Students were segregated from the graduate nurses both in residence and in the dining area. They were expected to defer to their superiors, even senior students, and were restricted in fraternizing with students in other classes. However, they did come up with creative ways to live with any restrictions. Oakley, "There were 10 or 11 of us [in our class] that would sit at the same table in the dining room." Whiteway, "Oh yes you'd mix with the other nurses. Now we didn't have a cafeteria, we had a dining room. You weren't really supposed to sit with them, you know, but you did it." Ashbourne, "I mean, it was stricter...you weren't supposed to mix with the crowd from the...like the probationers weren't supposed to mix with the [senior students]...and stuff like that." Bruce, "Among the beautiful memories that I have of my training days, was that beautiful dining room that we had and here was this great big class sitting at a big long table. We usually sat with our class. The graduates sat at smaller tables." Moakler, "...and senior nurses, if you saw a senior nurse going in the ward with a bedpan, you just rushed up and took the bedpan because that was...dirty duties would be your job! They were very strict, like, I had a girl in my class who had a sister a year ahead of her but they weren't allowed to mix. They weren't allowed to socialize...you weren't allowed to mix with the seniors. So they would meet downtown or something but they weren't allowed to be seen going down the lane together. [They wouldn't eat meals together in the cafeteria or anything like that]. The grads had one dining hall and the students had the other, and the 'probies,' as we were called, sat over in one corner and then the second years sat somewhere else and the third years sat somewhere else...a real class system." Avery, "We did not associate too much with the other class. Everybody knew his or her spot. [People in the senior class were senior]. Then at the same time we were above the junior class. When we went out we were Grace nurses, but in the hospital we held our position too." House, "When we would see a graduate go by, when we were in training, we would stand back and wait until she passed [because you were a student]." Story, "We were the lowest of the low on the list. We could not mix with the senior nurses and that really appalled me. I thought that nurses were very nice ladies but some of them were rough."

Under no circumstances would a student think to challenge the rules as demonstrated in Barron's story; "It [my lung] was collapsed when I finished training. When I went back to finish I only had this lung operating and that used to take a bit of energy (laughing)...especially when we weren't allowed to use the elevator. We had to use the stairs. I was running up the stairs this day, going all out and I was breathing heavy and panting and poor Sister she said, 'Miss Morry, what's wrong with you?' and I said (panting) 'Sister, I just had a pneumothorax done [at the San],' and it was 3:55 p.m. and I had to be on duty by 4:00 p.m. She said 'Miss Morry, my child, don't ever do that again, get on the elevator.' But we weren't allowed, we weren't allowed to use the elevators and I had to be on duty. No one could use the elevator unless you had a patient or something like that."

Although they did not challenge the status quo, neither were the students hindered by the rules and regulations. Often they came up with very creative ways of dealing with their circumstances. King, "There was a lot of comical things back then. I used to have to watch for Miss McGin. She was our matron of the home. They always made me do it because I never used to go out a great deal on dates in those days. I used to have to get at the head of the stairs and call out if somebody was down by the door and tell them to come in when it was safe. They depended on me for that."

Moakler, "We learned a lot. They were very strict with us. We were supposed to be ladies and when you went out in the daytime, you had to wear a hat and gloves. And going down that General Hospital lane, there were a lot of trees and it was just like you'd see for Halloween now with all the masks hung on the trees. All you'd see was hats and gloves down there, in the trees. So when you came back from downtown, you'd pick up your hat and gloves and went up to the office [you left the building with the hat and gloves on then left them in the trees until you returned]. You were a lady so you had to wear a hat and gloves...you were expected to be a lady. They were trying to teach you to be a lady. But, to me, that don't make a lady; a hat and gloves don't make a lady. You have to learn that on your own."

Like most things in life individuals learn to make choices about their circumstances, either adapt or let them get you down. These young women probably had plenty to complain about during their students days, however their stories clearly show they were quite capable of making the most of their situation. Therefore, it is not surprising that memories about residence and all things related to life as a student were vividly recalled and also evoked smiles and laughter some 50 years later.

PART 2:
Nursing Practice~Life After Graduation

Once they had graduated from nursing school, nurses were desperately required in the health care delivery system. As of 1931, nurses had to register with the Department of Health, if they wished to work as a registered nurse in the province. Only after 1937 or so, did they write a registration examination developed by the Department of Health. It was not mandatory to write these to work as a nurse but the majority of graduates did. Prior to this time nurses were not required to take any provincial examination only school examinations and these authorized them to work as a nurse. There was a professional association known as the Newfoundland Graduate Nurses Association that tried to establish standards for nursing but it had no legal status. Graduation from nursing school was the only prerequisite to taking on the full responsibilities of a nurse.

Once she became employed, the nurse was no longer under the control of the school, but her life did not change drastically. Often she still lived in a residence provided by the organization and worked long grueling hours. She was expected to provide whatever service was necessary whether she had experienced it in nursing school or not. The nurses' duties were frequently dictated by the medical doctor in the institution or community health department or, if there was no medical doctor, her duties were necessitated by the fact that she was the only health provider in the community and therefore did what she could with the resources available and the knowledge she had.

Nurses did not work solely for the money and in fact monetary rewards were often the lesser of their benefits. Instead they were rewarded with recognition as a professional. Others enjoyed the challenge and fulfillment that came from helping others. The nurse was respected because of her knowledge and skills and as such was frequently one of the leaders in a community. Often the nurse worked because she felt a calling to the profession and had a desire to help others. Whatever the particular job, the nurse often benefitted from emotional and social rewards as opposed to material compensation.

Health care delivery took place in the towns and the outports. Hospitals in Newfoundland were founded in the major economic centres such as Gander or the major ports such as St. John's, Corner Brook and Twillingate. The general hospitals dealt with all kinds of illness but also there were hospitals that were quite specialized such as the Merchant Navy Hospital, the Fever and the Sanatorium. Outside of the towns, outports were served by nurses sent there by the Health Department to work in cottage hospitals, by untrained midwives and by ships. The sea was a major part of peoples' lives so it is not surprising that ships such as the *Christmas Seal* (Tb ship) and the *Lady Anderson* (Public Health) were part of the health care system.

Our participants graduated anywhere from 1924 to 1949. In the 1930s some nurses were financially supported by such volunteer organizations as NONIA (Newfoundland Outport Nursing and Industrial Association). Whereas in 1949, Newfoundland had joined Canada and money became available to send nurses outside of the province for education. A nurse graduating early in this period would have been faced with a different world than a nurse graduating in 1949.

CHAPTER 5:

Getting a Job

"I didn't think I was doing anything spectacular. Now it frightens me. When I think back...it wasn't unusual, it was expected of you. I felt I was helping somebody and that's what I went into training for." Moakler (45)

Nurses had plenty of choice and at the mere suggestion of a friend or relative nurses were prepared to take or change jobs. (Upon graduation from nursing school, nurses seemed to have endless opportunities for jobs). There was a need to staff the hospitals in St. John's, cottage hospitals around the province and public health nurses were also needed everywhere. Jobs of every description were available. Some nurses chose jobs because of family circumstances while others chose jobs that fit with their personality. Most nurses interviewed are prime examples of self-directed, determined women, as are many Newfoundland women faced with lives of hard work. Many of these nurses should be seen as the unsung heros of the women's movement. Most were leaders in their communities or in their profession.

In the late 1930s Williams was living with her husband on Woody Island. "I was married a couple of years, he [her husband] said to me one day, 'Why don't you take up nursing?' Because they got no nurse here; only a midwife and she was after losing several babies and women, and so I phoned. Dr. Coxing was at Come-by-Chance and he got in touch with Dr. Miller...a public health doctor. And so they wired and asked me to meet them in Swift Current to talk over some business. I went and I met them and they wanted to know if I'd take up nursing in the Placentia Bay – for six months to relieve the pressure on Dr. Coxing for the summer. And, my dear, I was there for thirty-four years." Similarly, in 1948, Griffen was working part-time in Gander when she met her friend. "Miss Fitzgerald had worked in Botwood first when I came and she went over [to Corner Brook] to take over, to the new hospital that was being built. She said, 'The hospital is really short, Joan. The [new] hospital is not open. What about coming over and working in the old place.' And I said, 'Well, that's fine.' Because I was only relieving in Gander," and off she went to Corner Brook.

Newfoundland nurses were not intimidated by any nursing situation. Woodland found herself in Ottawa with her husband in 1965; "I just walked in off the street and went to the....I suppose she was Director of Nurses...and I said, 'Do you have any part-time work?' and she said, 'No but we have some full-time work.' And I said...well I just wanted to do nights 'cause I had four children. And she said, 'Oh, that would be marvelous!' She asked me what experience I had and I told her all the obstetrics experience I had and she said, 'Well, you know, that's not much good to us.' I said, 'No but sure I can learn.' And so she took me on...I went home and they phoned me and said, 'Come in to work tonight at 11:00 p.m.' I said, 'What? No orientation, no nothing.' 'Yes,' she said, 'We need someone on the surgical floor.' And I go up on the surgical floor. So that was my first experience there. I didn't know if I wanted to go back actually. No I didn't know...but I went back again after that and the girls I worked with were marvelous. And then I went down on the cardiac floor and the girls down there...I mean, they were something else – they were really, really nice. So I enjoyed working there." She worked there from 1965 to 1967 before coming back to Newfoundland.

Orientation: Individuals who entered nursing knew that they must be ready to adjust to the situation presented to them. The women we interviewed were courageous when faced with new experiences whether it was trampling though the bush, taking out teeth or delivering babies in unusual circumstances. It was rare that they would stay in one nursing job for their whole career, although a few did. Generally the nurses moved from widely varying nursing positions without complaint and coped with whatever the job presented. Throughout this period when the majority of these nurses worked, they rarely received any orientation to the organization or job they chose. However, there were some examples reported. A job orientation seemed to be limited to nurses coming from out of province or those moving north.

Although some nurses received an orientation of sorts to help with their new responsibilities, their expanded scope of practice went well beyond anything they had learned in nursing school. In most cases of nurses moving north, individuals took it upon themselves to get an orientation. It was not provided by the employer. Hutchings worked in St. John's for a short stint when she decided to work on the Northern Peninsula. She had little or no experience with deliveries. On her way she stopped off at the Bonne Bay Hospital where she stayed for two and a half months learning procedures she'd need up the coast. "People say, 'How can you do these kinds of things?' Like go off on your own and go off on the Northern Peninsula. When you're young, and I was twenty-four…the world is yours…you don't worry about anything. I packed up all my things in a trunk and had that shipped ahead. Now I left St. John's by train and got in Deer Lake [where I] stayed and the next day I went by taxi from Deer Lake to Bonne Bay. This was way back in 1949 and there was a road but it was a gravel road and it was not very good. And instead of going to Woody Point, we went to Lomond the next day by ferry and we came out by boat right away and came into Norris Point. And Dr. Murphy came down in his jeep and picked me up and took me into the hospital where I met [the other nurse]. There was only one road and the road was between Norris Point and Rocky Harbour. And Dr. Murphy…did a lot of deliveries for Rocky Harbour and Norris Point because I don't think they had a midwife there like I had down the coast. So, when he knew I was going on the coast and I was going to be working with him, he got me to observe deliveries and then he let me do a couple of deliveries. So I did two deliveries before I went on the coast; that's all I did. But the other thing he taught me, I had to pull teeth. So he showed me how he did it. I learned to infiltrate the Novocain around the tooth and then pull it out. I became very good at pulling teeth afterwards. And he taught me a little bit about suturing. So suturing and deliveries and pulling teeth were all learned in there."

Scope of Practice: Health care providers outside the urban areas were limited in number and the expectations of those nurses opting to work in these areas were high. In 1939 Giovannini (24) came to Newfoundland "…just before the last war. We were district nursing in England and were quite happy but there was the talk of the war and we were all issued gas masks. Apart from that, two of us thought we would like a change and we saw the advertisements in the paper about places in Newfoundland. There were small outports that had no medical help from either nurses or doctors and it appealed to us. We applied and we were told that we could go anywhere but we only worked in the small isolated outports. It appealed to us because we were used to working in the working class and the poor districts which I loved. Of course over here, we did not only have one place; we had eight or nine settlements to look after. First, we went to the Department of

Health in the Courthouse for orientation and that took about ten days. We went down there to learn what we had to do and also, we were horrified to learn that we had to learn dentistry and pull teeth."

As a new graduate Giffen took her first job in a cottage hospital; "I went to work in Botwood. And that was an experience because that's the cottage hospital (system), you know? It was quite large. I don't know how many patients we had, really and truly. It was quite a large place because it was...left by the army, the hospital was. I remember the first...second day, I was there and this man came in with his hand cut and so I called Dr. Rowe. I called him because he lived in what used to be a clinic next door. I said, 'There's a man here needs his hand sutured.' He said, 'What's the matter with you? Paralyzed?' I said, 'I'm only a nurse; I don't suture.' So he came over and he sutured the man's hand and then, after the man left, he brought me into the office and he said, 'Now you're just here, but I'll tell you, you can make up your mind whether you're going to stay or not,' he said, 'but there's only two of you, so you have to do the suturing, you have to pull teeth, you have to do all the deliveries except I'll come for the first delivery, the first baby, but after that I'll only come if you call me.' And he said, 'Then you have to do x-rays and blood.' Because they had no x-ray technician or blood, you know? We were master of all. And then he said, 'There's only two of you, so you decide between yourselves, one gives the anesthetic and the other assists at surgery.' So he said, 'If you want to do that, you can stay; if not, you know, you're no good here'." She had not learned any of these procedures in Nursing School.

The expectation of the nurse being ready to do whatever work necessary from day one was pervasive. Higgins worked on the dependants unit at the base hospital at Pepperell, where the military families were admitted. Her background was in the operating room but her duties there primarily involved deliveries; "Well, we weren't obstetrical nurses at the General, not at the time. We had two months. And I remember the...first time that I was on the dependents area of the building, and I came in the afternoon and there were two patients in labour, and they, the Americans, flung the fetoscope over to me. And I thought, well this is it! And I did it. I mean, things came at you and I did it. That was my prime responsibility even though I was...roaming the floor so I had a senior nursing assistant, or LPN (Licensed Practical Nurse) covering the floor for me...I knew who was down on that floor, probably about eight or ten post-delivery patients and so I checked on these and told her what to do and then I had to see these two deliveries. I hadn't done deliveries and I thought no way am I going to say…I don't know that much about obstetrics. Oh yes, I know it all! So I went through and then when I went in…the case room was familiar to me because I was an OR nurse, so I just did what he told me, what he wanted ready and we connected right away and so he started the delivery and I just started with some anesthetic there and I had everything ready and just went ahead."

No matter where one trained to be a nurse it seemed that they approached their work with the same attitude. Taylor was one of many British nurses who came to work on the isolated shores of Labrador in 1953: "I was always intending to go somewhere as a missionary. I was thinking of India actually. But while I was in Vancouver after my mother died, I decided I'd have to go somewhere else; I didn't know where or what. I went to Ottawa and a friend of mine mentioned the Grenfell Mission…so I started to make inquiries and got the forms and I still wasn't sure what I wanted to do. Eventually I did put in an application. I got accepted. And I set out from Montreal by boat." She landed in Blanc Sablon in September of 1953. The nurse who was there before met her and brought her to the nurses station in Forteau where she started work right away. "After she brought me in, she left about ten days later and left me to it. Well right at the first, she sent me up to Red Bay to do a medical thing. That's where I pulled my first teeth. But I did go to see a dentist in Ottawa before I left and he gave me a few pointers." Although Taylor didn't know what she would be faced with in Labrador, she tried to prepare for as much as she could anticipate.

Moakler relates her experience as a new graduate in public health; "I stayed on as a staff nurse for three months at the General. And then I went out on the southwest coast of Newfoundland on a hospital ship called the *Lady Anderson*, and worked for a year without a doctor. And we traveled from Grand Bank to François. I diagnosed, pulled teeth, treated, sutured…fools rush in where angels fear to tread. It was wonderful in the Operating Room in the cottage hospitals. We had doctors who were marvelous surgeons, and it was great! I didn't do a lot of scrub up work because I never liked OR work so I gave open needle, I gave the anesthetics. Yes, I know, no control, when you think about it. But, for the time, it wasn't unusual."

As time went along people realized that nurses needed an orientation when changing jobs even if they had lots of experience. By 1959 when

Roche decided to leave teaching at the General Hospital and join the Department of Health as Supervisor of Cottage Hospitals, South Coast Region, she was sent to a cottage hospital for experience; "I was there for a month to six weeks. It was an orientation." This was quite an extensive orientation before her move into her supervisory position. Although agencies attempted to orient staff to their role and responsibilities, in some cases it was better late than never. Woodland tells a funny story about her orientation when she started a part-time job at the Janeway Children's Hospital; "I went down to see the Director of Nursing down there to see if there was any part-time work and she said, 'Yes.' And that night I got a call, 'Come in.' And I went down. And I was working there about two years, I suppose, and I happen to do a day shift for some reason, and I believe the nurse's name was Mrs. Kent and she said, 'Oh you're a new one.' And I said, 'Yes.' She said, 'Oh I haven't had you for orientation yet.' I said, 'You're not likely to get me.' She said, 'Why?' I said, 'Because I've been here for two years!' And she said, 'Didn't you ever have orientation?' I said, 'No.' See they were so desperate, I guess, for people on nights."

A nurse today would expect an orientation when starting employment. Whether she is just out of nursing school or is a more experienced nurse changing jobs, some time would be set aside to review what was expected of her and what responsibilities she was to hold. The women who graduated from nursing school before 1950 were assumed to have adequate introduction to the profession to be able to handle any job. There was a prevailing notion that a nurse is a nurse and she should be prepared to adapt to anything and everything. This may have been true for nurses who stayed in the same institution where they graduated, but not so when they moved from this hospital. When possible they provided their own orientation. These young women worked courageously and functioned far beyond the scope of practice taught them in nursing school. They were often self-reliant and brave and didn't question authority. If the people in charge of the hospital or agency thought they were capable of doing the job, then they would do what was required.

CHAPTER 6 :
Nursing in Rural Newfoundland

"When you were out there you were pretty much on your own unless it was something very serious. I don't remember too many people ever being sent to St. John's other than terminally ill patients." Avery (45)

In rural Newfoundland nursing was delivered in nursing stations, cottage hospitals and by public health nurses throughout the province. Rural nursing was composed of any nursing taking place outside larger hospital settings with little or no access to services such as laboratories, x-rays and operating rooms. Nursing stations were small 'hospitals' in coastal communities which were manned solely by nurses, in many cases only one nurse. Cottage hospitals were very somewhat larger than the nursing station with a doctor on staff along with one or two nurses. Public health nurses often had no building to house their practice but worked out of their homes and were frequently on their own in their districts. Working conditions for all these nurses differed according to their proximity to St. John's.

Nursing in rural Newfoundland in the 1930s and 40s was an isolating experience. The nurse decided whether she could treat a health problem alone or if additional services were needed. This could mean something as simple as consulting a doctor in a larger center, or it could mean transporting the patient to another community at a time when provincial transportation was not easy. Ultimately, the nurse had to feel confident her decision was the best possible solution and had to be accountable for any decisions made. In many respects she functioned similarly to the nurse practitioner of today.

Nursing Stations: The most isolated form of rural nursing was the nursing station. In northern Newfoundland and Labrador, nurses worked for the International Grenfell Association which opened its first nursing station in 1908 in Forteau, Labrador. Most of the nurses who went to nursing stations in Labrador and northern Newfoundland at that time were from out of the country, often British nurses, young women out to have an adventure. Some stayed longer but most stayed for the two years required by their contract and then returned to England. It was unusual for Newfoundland trained nurses to work in these areas. Penney and Ashbourne indicated that in the late 1940s and early 1950s, the nurses working at St. Anthony were mostly American, likely recruited by NONIA.

The focal point for the Grenfell Association and health care in northern Newfoundland was the Grenfell Hospital in St. Anthony. This hospital received emergency patients and served as a source of advice and information to nurses in remote nursing stations. Doctors from there would travel out into the communities for clinics and visit patients referred by the nurse. Nurses, who were based in coastal communities, lived in and worked out of the nursing stations. These nursing stations served as their home and as a hospital for patients. In these stations the nurse was the only person with any education in health and she worked with very limited resources.

Taylor came to southern Labrador as a missionary which was unusual. She was located in Forteau on the southern Labrador coast and was responsible for communities from there to Red Bay about 40 miles north. "They tried to persuade everybody (patients) to come up to the nursing station. There were some local midwives who were local women but not real midwives. The people would stay in different homes if they had friends here and then some of them would stay at the nursing station. We tried to get them to stay there. This was just during the days when travels were by boat and dog team. When the road came through we didn't always have the same problem. That was about '56. Twice a year the doctor from St. Anthony came. They came in the little mission boats in the fall and in the summer and during the winter everybody came by airplane." When the road was put through to Red Bay the people had better access to health care facilities.

Nurses in the stations also traveled to isolated communities to bring health care to the people. Taylor recalls such a visit to Red Bay, "About 50 miles...I went down on one of the coastal boats. I came back by motor boat. I was going to do a clinic. Clinics in all the different communities were in somebody's house. [The previous nurse] told me which houses we went to. They probably volunteered. It was done before I got here. [I saw] children, antenatals, anything; the same as you would in a clinic. Earaches and sore throats and chest infections and measles. We had medications. It was given to treat our own patients. I had to diagnose and treat. In antenatal, you made sure they were healthy. Immunizations sure. And we'd do home visits when we went out. Then I went to the next community which was where people went during the summer for fishing. It's behind Red Bay, a couple of minutes by boat."

Because these nurses were the only people in the community who were knowledgeable about health care they were never off duty. Taylor, "I remember going up to Lanse au Loop for a concert and in the middle...somebody came up to me and said, 'Nurse what's this thing on my wrist?' It was a lump or something. And I remember the nurse's aide who was there when I first came, she went to get married and at the wedding, somebody decided to fall into the brook and nearly get drowned. So I got called out, of course."

Labrador and northern Newfoundland presented many challenges to the nurses working in these isolated areas. Penney, who worked with Community Health in St. John's, volunteered to go to St. Anthony and transport a patient who needed to be admitted to the hospital in St. John's. She traveled there in a small plane and became stranded when the plane had mechanical difficulties; "In St. Anthony once navigation closed in the fall, they didn't see anybody again 'til the spring, so it was great to have the plane come in. We landed on the ice and everybody in the whole community was down because I could see them coming. You know, it was great! And then actually he couldn't get the plane off for a couple of days. We were there for almost two weeks before we got out of it."

During her time in St. Anthony, Penney had an opportunity to meet one of the English nurses in a nursing station; "She was an English nurse. There were English and American [nurses] mostly there. But they were wonderful girls because they worked hard and under all sorts of poor conditions. Well because I was down there for two weeks, they said to me, 'Would you like to come across to Hooping Harbour? We're going across by komatik [dogsled].' They had their nursing station over there. And they had to bring some supplies over there for her. She had a direct line with a doctor there and she would call. I thought that girl was really great. She had amputated two toes, but it wasn't hard to amputate them because gangrene had set in and they were falling off anyway. She was really busy there [in] Hooping Harbour. She was assigned there from Grenfell [Hospital]."

Cottage Hospitals: In 1936, the Department of Health opened cottage hospitals in an effort to organize delivery and improve the standards of health care throughout the province particularly in rural areas. These were generally small but were different from nursing stations in that cottage hospitals had a doctor on staff along with nurses. The doctor was definitely in charge but the nurse was responsible for the day to day operations of the hospital and also did most of the patient care. Nurses in cottage hospitals were the live-in staff and like nurses in nursing stations were on-call more often than not.

Roche was employed as a supervisor in the cottage hospital system. "We had to work eighteen cottage hospitals at a time and we had it divided up into three each [per supervisor]. I did the South Coast, someone else, the Northeast, and somebody else did the West Coast. We had to check out everything in these hospitals; we had to check problems that nurses were having with doctors and sort them out. Some of the hospitals only had a few nurses and they worked very hard. There were usually only two doctors there." She explained the nursing structure in the Department of Health at the time, "There was the director, an associate director, and eventually, we became assistant directors." Although the nursing supervisor did not have a great deal of influence in the working of the department they were responsible for most of the staffing in the hospitals. Roche, "We had very little to do with the secretary's employment or the people that worked with them. We employed the nurses and when we could, we interviewed. The nursing assistants were usually employed directly by the nurse in charge of the hospital." The supervisors were also responsible for the midwives in the area. Roche, "I only ever got to see two or three of them. Because they were all in little coves that the boats could not get into."

Griffen describes what it was like to work in Botwood Cottage Hospital; "But then, you worked every morning…well, you went to work at 8:00 a.m but you lived in the hospital. There were only two nurses. Every second night, you were on call. So, that night, you couldn't go to bed until 1:00 a.m. or 2:00 a.m. depending on what was going on. And all the medications were given out because we had nurse's aides in those days but, they only gave bedpans and did stuff like that. And if anything came in the night like anybody in labour or an accident or anything, you had to get up. But you still had to go to work the next day whether you got in bed or not. [This happened], quite often. Every day and every second night was your call. While the nurses were in surgery the nursing assistants would look after the patients." The interdependence of the groups was obvious.

Avery who worked in Old Perlican relates a similar story; "We had one cook for the hospital, our water was brought by gravity from a pond above the hospital, and we hired ladies from Old Perlican to come in on Mondays. We did not have a washing machine so they had to do the laundry by scrubbing the clothes on boards. That is the way it was. We actually lived in the Cottage Hospital upstairs. The other nurse and myself each had a room and we shared a common bathroom with the three nursing assistants. One of the assistants would do the night duty, and when women would go into labour, [she] would come and call us. I've delivered babies in my dressing gown. The doctor was close by, only being across the road, but he was not always available. There was a nurse in charge and when that nurse was gone, the second nurse was in charge and they did whatever had to be done."

Hutchings worked in Rocky Harbour Cottage Hospital in preparation for being the lone community nurse in Cow Head. "We really didn't have any time off. One of us was on call every night. And maybe we'd have Saturday afternoon off or Sunday but we never spent the night [away from the hospital]…maybe go for a walk or you'd go out to the store. I used to do a fair amount of walking." Life for a nurse in a cottage hospital was demanding with little free time. The community depended on the nurses to be available whenever needed and didn't imagine that they would need personal time. Avery, "They'd get in such a state and they think there is nobody there to do it. It had been near Christmas and I was gone into Old Perlican to buy some decorations for the hospital. When I got back, they were there at the door and I thought for sure I was going to be fired!" The nursing assistants and patients felt deserted because she wasn't immediately available.

Much of the work done in cottage hospitals depended on the skills and interests of the medical staff, the staffing available, the degree of isolation of the hospital and the resources available. Like their colleagues in the bigger centers, the nurses in cottage hospitals also performed multiple roles when caring for patients. In Rocky Harbour there was no way to transport patients and the staff had to take care of all patient care. Hutchings, "We had two rooms for obstetrics. We had an Operating Room. And downstairs we had a really cramped outpatients and in the outpatients was Dr. Murphy's office. And outside of his office we had a great big long counter with all the medications on it and that's where the nurse worked.

He would see the patients and then he'd send them out to you with a little slip of paper and whatever medications they had to have. We had to fill the medications and sing out to them [the patients] and they'd come and get it. He would try to do the ones with x-rays before 11:00 o'clock and then he'd always have a break for a cup of tea or go upstairs in the sitting room, the nurse's sitting room upstairs, and we'd have a cup of tea and maybe a sandwich. And then he'd come down and do his x-rays himself and read them and come back and call the patients in again. And he did a lot of deliveries." Botwood was isolated, but there was some communication with the hospital in Grand Falls. As Griffen stated, "Dr. Rowe did big surgery. And even Dr. Strong, from Grand Falls, used to come down and they'd do hysterectomies and bones and anything that occurred. Dr. Rowe would do it, Noonan gave the anesthesia and I elected to assist."

Avery worked in Old Perlican, nearer St. John's and its larger medical centers. "Normally, there were eleven patients. You could probably have 12 or 13 because you could put in two more beds. They did a lot of operations at Old Perlican Cottage Hospital. We pulled teeth and did everything. We sterilized our instruments and made up trays. I was a scrub nurse all the while I was there, I put in every effort for every operation that was there."

The cottage hospital system required that families pay a yearly fee for medical care given in hospital but drugs, maternity and dental care cost extra. Hutchings, "Now in the cottage hospital system, they saw the doctor for free and it didn't cost them anything to have x-rays or anything like that, but the medications, in a lot of cases, they paid for unless they were on welfare and then we'd pay for it and mark it in." The decision to access health care could hinge on the ability to pay. Avery shared a story of how the inability to pay impacted on the lives of the people. "This lady went into labour in Old Perlican. I requested that she be brought in and he [her husband] said 'No. It would cost too much money.' So he called me out. When I got out there she was in heavy labour and she was bleeding a lot. I brought her in and got her into the case room and cleaned her up so I could see what we were doing. I saw that it was placenta previa. I had her there a little while and I was trying to get the doctor. It was after 10:00 o'clock by the time that I got her in. The phones were cut off at 10:00 o'clock and I could not get any phone-calls until 8:00 o'clock in the morning. When I got her in I gave her a shot of Morphine and prayed that it would hold her until morning, but it didn't, of course. She woke up about 1:00 or 2:00 o'clock and delivered immediately and it was a dead infant.

Everything was separated and the sac wasn't even broken. I was so hopeful that maybe the baby was alive. It was such a beautiful baby. The next morning I got a hold of the doctor and we got her fixed away in the bed. At this time she was aware that the baby was stillborn. I believe that the baby was dead when I got out there the night before, because I could see something but I did not know what it was. Anyway, I told the doctor what I had done and that I had sat with her. He fixed everything off and that was it." This story provides insight into both the difficult conditions under which nurses worked and the impact of not having ready access to health care but it also shows the measures nurses were prepared to take in order to care for their patients.

Griffen was also expected to do visits by boat. "We were in Botwood one night, they sent a boat [because there was] a woman in labour somewhere and I went with Dr. Rowe. We steamed for an hour and a half wherever we went and you'd blow when you get into a harbour, the captain blows to get somebody to come out. So this man arrived out in the little boat and he said to Dr. Rowe, 'Doctor' he said, 'the man above got here before you.' So Dr. Rowe said, 'Well done, Jesus!' and turned around and came back. I said, 'Dr. Rowe, you know you're going in to check her.' He said, 'No. She delivered. That's all. We'll go back to Botwood.'

The hard work and long hours fostered interdependence and comradery among the staff of a cottage hospital. They relied on each other. Avery describes it this way: "It was a great experience to be there. It was good being a nurse. We were close." Hutchings drew a similar conclusion, "I thoroughly enjoyed it when you got into it. Yes and because we were such a small group there, it was like a family."

The cottage hospital system served the Newfoundland people for almost 50 years but eventually they were turned into health clinics under the auspices of the hospital board in the region. Roche noted the passing of the era of the cottage hospital "...in the 80s. They did not close them, they put them under another place. Like, Grand Falls took over Harbour Breton, and Corner Brook took over Burgeo."

Public Health Nursing: Before 1934 public health was run by volunteers who were generally the elite of Newfoundland women. One example was the Newfoundland Outport Nursing and Industrial Association (NONIA) started in 1920. Through the sale of knit goods, money was raised to finance the work of nurses assigned to rural districts in Newfoundland. Another volunteer group was the Child Welfare Association established by a group of women in St. John's. It provided services to mothers, babies and children up to the age of five in St. John's and surrounding communities. Godden, "I think it was '39 when I went to Child Welfare to work. I think it was soon after I finished. It was run by a committee of ladies who belonged to the town. They weren't nurses or anything. Lady Outerbridge was one; she was President of the Association. I suppose that was civic minded. We'd get our birth list from the government, and everybody [born] in the town, we'd have to get a card for them and we visited. And there was five or six nurses. We used to go to the homes and do the immunizations but we had clinics outside like Petty Harbour and Bay Bulls...and Portugal Cove and we had clinics and people would bring their babies to the clinics and have their needle and see the doctor and all that. We also had a children's clinic – usually up to five years of age but, if they were six, we'd see them."

In 1934, the Department of Public Health and Welfare established a nursing service, district nurses, to take over functions at volunteer organizations such as Child Welfare. In 1937, the department established a second nursing division, the public health nursing service and freed up the district nurses to do maternity and home care. This was the beginning of community health nursing around the province as we know it today. Likely this was Government's attempt to set some standards for delivery of community nursing services throughout the island. In 1941 both these divisions were amalgamated.

While all nurses working in Public Health were employed by the Department of Health, there were distinct differences in the work of the public health nurses in St. John's as compared to those working in communities in rural parts of the island. That is not to say that either group was any more or less important than the other, just that the span of their responsibilities was different as well as the geographic boundaries of their practice. Nurses working in St. John's had access to resources such as supplies, doctors, an office, and hospitals whereas rural community health nurses, depending on location, often were the sole health care providers who made do with whatever was available. Nurses in St. John's also didn't have the transportation challenges of nurses in rural Newfoundland.

Public Health (Rural Areas): Public health nurses in rural Newfoundland traveled under risky and severe conditions to care for their patients. In 1935 Williams entered public health in Placentia Bay; "I enjoyed it but I went through an awful lot. At first when I got there, 'twas all boats – not covered-in boats, just the boat and sometimes they'd throw a sail over me where the water wouldn't go over me. And then after a few more years, they had a covered-in boat. I had four places. I had Woody Island, Bar Haven, Davis Cove, and Monkstown and, when I'd get to Davis Cove to get to Monkstown, I had to go by horse and buggy or sometimes I had to walk it – that was eight miles. I'd go out to Davis Cove in boat; that would be an hour and a half getting out there. And sometimes you wonder if you were ever going to live to get there – it would be so stormy. My husband's brother had a boat. But then, if they wanted me in Bar Haven, they'd come down in their own boat for me. Many a time going to Bar Haven, we ran up on a rock. The boat would be stuck up on a rock and, here I'd be, up looking down at the water." Hutchings on the Northern Peninsula traveled about in much the same way, taking whatever means of transportation available; "When I started to give the immunizations, I did Sally's Cove in the summer because that was the only time I could get there. From Sally's Cove to Green Point, I'd go by boat. But St. Paul's and Parson's Pond, I did those in the spring and the fall. And, if I couldn't get there by boat, I walked." For the public health nurse the opening of a road in her assigned area brought about big changes in health care delivery. Hutchings, "There's like two parts of nursing: when I was isolated and after the road came. We were isolated until '62, you couldn't really plan things. But after the bridge went across St. Paul's and there was a good bridge across Parson's Pond going down to Portland Creek, even though it was only a gravel road, you could go and you could say now I'm going to do a set thing."

The geography of most rural districts was large compared to St. John's and transportation was very difficult. Often the nurse had to rely on the generosity of the people in each community that she visited for food and lodging. Giovannini in the early 1940s had to travel on long trips to get to her patients. She would stop at homes along the way to get food and was grateful for whatever was offered. "You had to go into any house that would give you a meal. That is right. These people had seal soup and I never tried it before but I ate it and I was still alive." Hutchings, "Every place you went, you had somewhere there to stay. Nearly every place had someone with a spare room. After I was in awhile, when I'd go to different places I made arrangements with the Department of Health that I would pay them. And pay for my meals."

Nurses were called upon to do extraordinary things in extraordinary circumstances but with an attitude pervasive in nurses of that generation they adapted to the circumstances without question. Williams, "I delivered a baby in the boat going from Woody Island to Swift Current, off Rattling Brook, on the Mainland. It was called Woody Island Mainland. It happened there was a house [on the boat] and she was down in the house. So when I knew she was in labour, I called out to her husband; he was steering the boat with the big rudder tiller wheel 'I'll go in here in the little cove' he said 'and anchor and see what's going to take place.' And that's what he did. My dear we were tossing up and down and I delivered that baby girl. I had no facilities [at the clinic] so he took me on to Swift Current and I went on to Come-by-Chance Hospital." Nurses had to be very self reliant and often circumstances required they make judgements that they felt were in the best interests of their patients but outside the rules. Giovannini, "That is one time when you could use your own discretion and it worked. Well, I left her all night. You see we were not supposed to give any Morphine or anything like that but I did give that to this woman and let her rest. We delivered the baby the next day. If I had kept on with her then, she would have been torn to pieces."

The daily routine of the public health nurse ranged from fairly routine baby clinics to the extraordinary. Usually there was quite a volume of work which included a variety of responsibilities. Hutchings, "I had a clinic in Cow Head on Monday from 10:00 a.m. to 12:00 p.m. and 2:00 p.m. to 4:00 p.m. Tuesday I went outside the district. I went to Parson's Pond two Tuesdays a month; St. Paul's one Tuesday a month, and Sally's Cove and Green Point the next Tuesday. On Wednesday, I had ordinary clinic in the morning and I had antenatal clinic in the afternoon. This was in Cow Head and mothers in Cow Head would bring their babies the same time as I had antenatal clinic. On Thursday was my school day because I had a lot of schools. I had nine schools. Every term I had to do rapid classroom which was checking their heads for lice and nits and their hands for scabies and that was very important because we did have it. You'd have to write out notes and the ones you picked up with any nits had to stay home and then they had to come back to me and make sure they were okay before I sent them back to school again. In grade one, I would do a complete physical. I would do the height and weight...and their ears. I did ears by whispering. I'd turn them one side and I'd say 'house, mouse' and they could pick up what it was and you'd be surprised how many children you could pick up with hearing defects from doing the whispering. And then I did eyes. I did the eye chart…hearing and eyes. And I could tell if the child was underweight by their weight and by their height, okay? Anyhow on Thursdays was my day for schools and I was really busy. Except for one Thursday a month when I did my report and that took me all day. Now if I got a child in kindergarten who was underweight, well then I would contact the parent…I'd contact the parents and I'll get them on Maltovol or I'd see them again within a month's time. And I would do the mothers by going into the home because I found that by going into the home you could see the situation. If you're in a place very long, after a while you'll know if the father is well…how they're doing financially…if they got gardens…or things like this."

Merrigan, "They used to call it district nurse, but it was all the same. I was in Avondale and St. Joseph's. We used to visit [the patients] and see how they were. If they had any sores or anything we would dress them and tell them what to do and about the medicine. Miss Squires [the supervisor] was in St. John's. She used to visit us. If you had an emergency, you had to call the doctor. We visited schools. We gave them their needles, checked for head lice, and made sure that their tonsils were not enlarged. I remember one time I went down to Athens Beach to take out a man's tooth, and no way could I get it out. But another friend of mine, Miss O'Flaherty, was down in St. Mary's and she helped me with it. She had training for that where I did not. I was ashamed to meet him [the patient] after! I remember in Avondale, they used to come for Cod Liver Oil and I used to give it to them. Well, I heard after that they were giving it to their horses!"

Home visits were also a part of the public health nurses daily routine but there was nothing routine about the care given each patient nor the relationships that formed between the nurses and their patients. Avery describes one of the patients she cared for as a public health nurse, "There was this man who had cancer of the pancreas. He had a catheter in and assumed that he was going to have this catheter out. But as time went on, he felt he was getting worse and wondered when the catheter was going to come out. He would always ask me when it was coming out and I could not tell him because it was up to his doctor. So, one day I said to him, 'Matt, I don't think that they will take out the catheter, this is your lifeline.' [The catheter went] into his gallbladder; it was bile that was coming out. After I told him that, he looked at me and considered it for a little while and then I believe he understood, and he nodded. After that, when I would go in to change his dressing and wipe around the catheter, he asked me about having it changed. I informed him to ask his doctor. Apparently, they did change it but they really did not want to. I knew that they were not going to do it anymore if this did not work. Anyway, when I would go in to change his dressing, he would be throwing questions at me hand over fist, that I would not know how to answer. When I would leave after an hour of talking to him, I would feel very drained because his last words would always be, 'Don't tell Enid.' Enid was his wife who was always right behind the door waiting for me to come out and ask me what went on. Anyway, I would have to tell her so much and ask her not to tell him. But we worked it all out and toward Christmas he wanted to sell his tools and buy whatever he could for his kids. That did happen and they had a really good Christmas but he was really sick. On Old Christmas Day, January 6, I went in to do his dressing and realized that the catheter was out. Of course, I lifted the catheter with the forceps and he looked at me and nodded his head. He died that night. It was just like he was part of my day; when he died I had nothing to do."

The nurses' commitment to their work and patients often meant that family life took a back seat to work. Williams was the only nurse in the area and like many public health nurses around Newfoundland was torn between the patient and her own famil; "I was out this night Christmas Eve. I never got home before 2:00 o'clock Christmas morning, I had delivered a baby. And when I got into bed, my husband said, 'Now, this is Christmas. You're not leaving this house Christmas Day.' I said, 'Okay.' We were having breakfast and he said, 'Don't you forget what I told you this morning. If anyone comes for you today, you're not going to go with them. We got a chicken in the oven and a girl there looking after it, so you're staying home.' I said, 'All right boy, I'll do what you tell me to do.' I was eating my breakfast and my table went along by the window on Woody Island, and I looked over the hill. And I saw this boat coming in to the wharf and I didn't say anything, and by and by I saw this man coming up over the hill walking in towards the house. I said, 'Beaton [her husband], look there's a man coming down.' And I said, 'You know, there's something wrong for him to come Christmas Day.' He said, 'Don't forget what I said.' So anyway, a rap come to the door and I went out and he said, 'I'm from Bar Haven.' I knew who he was. He said, 'My wife is dying, nurse, I'm sorry to come.' I'll never forget what he said with tears rolling down over his face, my dear! 'I'm sorry,' he said 'I had to come, nurse. I knows you can to do something.' I said, 'Come in, sir.' I said, 'Beaton, this man says his wife is dying and he wants me to come. What am I going to do?' My dear! He jumped up from the table. He says, 'Ethel, when duty calls her danger, be never walking there. Pack your bag and go.' I saved her. She had a four-month baby [premature]. And he got frightened because she was bleeding. But the baby was only four months...so…[it died]. So that's where I spent me Christmas Day in Bar Haven. And about 4:00 o'clock in the evening, my husband and his brother and his wife came up in their motorboat to see what was happening. And we went across the Cove to another house and went in there and that's where we had our Christmas supper. And I had my Christmas dinner at this woman's mother in law. And she was a cook for the priest in Placentia before she married and, my dear, she had chicken, stuffed, and I had the biggest kind of Christmas dinner!"

Supplies needed by the nurses in rural areas were generally stored in the nurse's home. Merrigan kept her supplies "…just in a bag that we carried around. We had a shelf whereever we boarded." Avery's supply storage changed over time; "When I went to Seal Cove there was no office. When I asked them for a file cabinet they told me to put my things in a trunk. So, I started off with a trunk and a taxi. The trunk would contain files, a book for keeping a record of my work on a daily basis, and a few pages for my travel expenses. We had to give a report every month. At that time, it was just building up a public health system on the shore." In comparison Hutchings was lucky because she had a clinic; "Now the clinic we had was built by the people, in a building by itself. It had an oil stove and it had canvas on the floor. I had a daybed in the main part of it. I had a waiting room with sort of a bench all the way around built into the wall for people to sit on. No heat. I had a small room that contained the drugs, had a chair with the dental rest on it. I had a washstand, for washing my hands, and a towel rack. I had buckets in the back part for bringing in water from the well. I think that the oil drum was in the clinic in the back. They had shelves in there with things like dressings and pads and extra medications and (equipment) for pulling teeth."

Like their counterparts working on the coast or in cottage hospitals, the public health nurse was also expected to be available whenever she was needed without expectations of overtime pay or time off. Merrigan describes patients going to her home, "They would come but they were not supposed to. There was an understanding that we could not be called in the middle of the night unless it was necessary. But I never did turn them away." Nurses were visited for all kinds of problems or to get preventative medications or advice.

Although there was poverty throughout Newfoundland, people who lived in the outports had gardens, and access to the fishery, and hunting. Giovannini shared her perspective of rural life when she was a public health nurse, "But I did go to a place one time and the old lady took me in for the night. Of course, she had bologna and that is about all the poor old thing had. She had it again [the next morning] but then I would not want them to know because I did appreciate it very much. They were very, very kind. [But] the people were not as badly off as some may think. Everybody had their gardens and they had hens and sheep. They would get moose and things like that. They never went hungry; they had their own vegetables and would pick berries. The people were very, very good. They would always bring you some berries, a partridge, or a rabbit."

Public Health (Urban): Public health nurses in St. John's functioned quite differently from their counterparts in the rural areas. Community Health in St. John's was divided into districts which included the surrounding communities such as Portugal Cove. The nurses had greater access to resources, doctors and hospitals. They did not have the same span of responsibilities or the same commuting problems as nurses in rural Newfoundland although very often they did encounter the same health problems particularly in the schools.

Avery, "I came into St. John's and I worked with Public Health around St. John's. We would go down by streetcar...down onto Water Street. We would sign in when we got there, pick up our bags, supplies, and so many nurses would get in a car and we would be put off at a certain place. Sometimes you would be put off at a school for a day and do a few things or dressings along the way. You spent most of the time walking. I didn't really like that but I did learn St. John's." Penney, "I really enjoyed Public Health. I did, I must say. Our offices were down behind the old Newfoundland Hotel. That's where Public Health was situated in those days. And we did five days a week then, and we did night-call. We did night-call in our turn which came up every couple of weeks, every two or three weeks, because there wasn't that many of us in town. And otherwise you did eight-hour shifts. It was great! Oh yes, that was real living. And we could come home for our lunch, and that was wonderful."

Public health nurses working in St. John's faced the poverty that was prevalent around the island but they also faced different social issues than nurses in rural Newfoundland. The city presented its own unique challenges. Moakler was a public health nurse for several districts in the city; "They were so poor and, I wouldn't say illiterate; I don't think that's the word to use, but there was a lot of incest and you had to be so careful. I did get involved in a Family Court thing when I was there. I had a call one night and this mother was screaming on the phone and she said, 'Come right away. My baby is bleeding.' So I got up there and this mother was about seven months pregnant I guess...the husband, or her second husband, came home with a few drinks in. I presume he wanted some sexual relationship with her and she refused so he grabbed the three-year old and stepped on her. So I ended up in court with that one. And it wasn't very nice from what I remember. Last going off...when I came back to public health, I made a few calls [to those same districts] to some of the nurses and it's so different; everyone there is so educated now and the homes are so beautiful."

Penney, "I did VD (Venereal Diseases) clinic for two years, and we had to go out and get our contacts. Some would come in and we'd treat them with Penicillin. We had a doctor there. And also in that clinic we did mostly all the different inoculations, for smallpox and that sort of thing. I don't know why they put it in the VD clinic but that's where it was."

Similarly the nurses' stories reflected the poverty that existed in urban Newfoundland. Many of the poorer women delivered their babies at home in terribly unhygienic surroundings. Penney relates some of the measures used for deliveries. "If they'd come to anti-natal clinic you had a better chance of giving them a little bit of education. Telling them what to get...they'd sew together newspapers for pads for underneath while they were delivering. And then we always had a few [pads] in our bag; we brought our obstetrical bag with us. We always brought some soup and whatnot because sometimes there was no food in the house to give them after they had their delivery."

Public health nursing in St. John's had its routine but the nurse didn't work in the same isolation as did rural nurses. The nurses had each other as well as a support system provided by the Department of Health. There was more use of shift work and nurses were required to be on call the same as cottage hospital nurses they just didn't live in. They had access to a car and driver if they were called out at night. The call for the public health nurse at night was directed through the hospital so the nurse always had access to the doctor, if needed, but this was unusual. The public health nurse in St. John's worked very independently and had the authority to make decisions about the treatment interventions. Moakler, "We were on call overnight and, you might be on call every second night and you still had to go to work the next day. We did a lot of home deliveries then so we would have to go with the home deliveries. We had a driver. There were several drivers in the Department of Health and we'd get a call at our home…the people who would need us would call the hospital; the hospital would call our home. We'd go down to our office to pick up the emergency bag and go off with the driver who came for us, and then we'd come back. It could be 2:00 or 3:00 o'clock in the morning, it didn't make any difference. And then we got up and went to work the next day and never thought anything about it." Barron, "Now, I was only hired on for five months, and we did call. We did two…one night was the first call, and another night you did second call, so you were on call for two nights a week, but you rarely got called in on the second call, but you were there in case of an assistant. And you did call on the weekends, some things like that. Now you didn't get paid extra for that." Penney, "And well we did the schools. We had general clinic, and the patients would come in. But then you had a lot of home visiting, and home deliveries, and they were mainly in the night. Or sick babies at night, and you made your own decisions. You had to decide whether you needed a doctor or not, or whether you need to take them to the hospital or not, but you could do that yourself. And you could also almost diagnose because you could give Penicillin and that, without an order. But you had to, because we didn't have the doctors. And we'd follow-up the next day."

Dewling worked with public health from the mid 50s to the mid 60s as a school nurse. "I did home visits and connected with the schools. We did all of the pre school exams, we checked the children to make sure they were healthy and in school and if they were not in school, we went to the home to see how they were. We had a lot of problems in the schools then with impetigo and lice; there was not a morning that you went in that you did not receive a call from one of the schools to go and check this out."

On occasion the nurse would consult with the doctor before going on call and, if he deemed it necessary, he would accompany the nurse but this was rare. Barron, "I was called one night and…around 12:00 o'clock. Now one of the good things about that…there was always good things…we had a drive. Someone would pick you up and drive you, which was quite different from today. Now up there, there was no telephone service or lights or anything when you're going out into the woods. So that night, when I got the information, someone got a phone somewhere out there and phoned us. This lady was breathing...she had the symptoms of a coronary. That's what she sounded like. So you kinda had to diagnose...well you diagnosed. So I called down to the General because there was always a doctor on call, and I thought before I get up there and there's no phone in that house and I wouldn't know where to find a phone and have to go God knows where to get a phone. I called down and Dr. Ring...he's on call and he's a young doctor from Ireland and I explained the symptoms of this lady and asked him what he would suggest, and he said 'You come down here and I'll go with you.' I would have been up there alone. Even with the doctor and driver it could be scary finding the patient's home. There was a lady, she said she would have a white bandana on, or a scarf, or something on her head, and she would meet us on the road, which she did. And then we had to follow her. Like you're going in the woods too, that's what it was like. I wouldn't want to do that again. I really was happy to have two men with me...because the driver would come up and pick you up. They were really good. So you walked up to the woods and then you got into this little house. Now that's the type of thing we did."

It also fell to the community health nurses to fly out into the smaller communities and collect patients who needed to be flown back into St. John's or to accompany patients for treatments in larger centers on the mainland. Barron explains what such a flight entailed, "I did a couple of mercy flights, left on a little plane, one engine plane, on Quidi Vidi and we used to go to Corner Brook." Penney, "And then, too, we did a lot of mercy flights. But now they were earlier on, as I think back, because I remember doing mercy flights and having to go down the cape. A mercy flight is what they called it. For instance, the lady I brought up had a brain tumor...and she was from Torbay somewhere. I took her to the Neuro in Montreal because we didn't have any facility here for neurosurgery at that time. And then I went one time to St. Anthony and we went down in January and hoping to get back in two days, at the most, and I ended up down there 12 days because of the weather and we had a little Piper Cub is what I went in, a two-seater, and we got down there and we couldn't get out of it. But that was to bring up a tuberculosis patient who was very ill and who had hemorrhaging and what not and they were sending her up to the San, but we only got back as far as Gander because he cancelled the flight there. One of the pontoons…oh, he had all kinds of trouble with the plane! But so we got on the train from there and came in and brought her to the San, and she had what they used to call 'millery Tb' in those days. So she died actually. This was before Confederation."

Griffen also did mercy flights; "Yeah, when I was in St. John's, I used to go out and pick up passengers…patients from around the coast. It used to take off from Octogon Pond in St. John's. The pilot would have the plane but I'd be the nurse who would be taking the patients back. And you ran in some little places and, honest to God, you'd think you were from outer space. The whole crowd would be out staring at you. It would be just when they needed somebody to go out and pick up a patient. All around the coast, everywhere. I remember coming in to Gander one night; we were going to land in Gander, and it was dark. You couldn't land after dark, and I remember the pilot said to me, 'What are we going to do with her, the woman?' I said, 'I got nothin' to give her, but I'm more worried about what you're going to do with us.' Because, he said, 'Have you ever been to Crosbie's Cabins?' and I said, 'No.' He said, 'I think that's where we're going to have to go tonight.' I said, 'Well I'm more worried with what you're going to have to do with me; I think I'd like to land in Gander tonight, myself!' We did make it to Gander but it was an experience! That would have been…let me see now…it was about '61 or '62. The plane from St. John's would pick them up and bring them mostly to Gander, the nearest hospital. They'd be very sick, half dead when you picked them up. Sometimes there were maternity [patients] that were having complications but not ready to be delivered."

Public health nurses were well received and respected in the community. As the public health nurse moved around her district she was easily recognized by her uniform. Avery, "In the winter we had a suit with a navy blue jacket, white blouse and a skirt. While we were doing clinics we had white aprons we would wear. In the summer for a while, we had light blue dresses and later, navy. They were rather nice and lightweight. We wore hats during most of my time; the last summer hat that we had, nobody could wear it. It was really round like a little pancake on your head. Everyone knew who I was."

Nursing in the community was challenging and varied in scope whether it was public health nursing in the rural or urban areas, a nursing station or a cottage hospital. This group of women had a clear notion of their role,

'to serve their patients' and did so without question. They were independent, versatile women, committed to their work and the people. Their
recollections tell of the measures they were willing to take to care for
their patients. But what choice did they have? As many stated, 'There
wasn't always a doctor.' Without these nurses, many areas and people
around the island would have had no access to health care. Their stories
clearly demonstrate the importance of the nurse to health care delivery in
Newfoundland and Labrador.

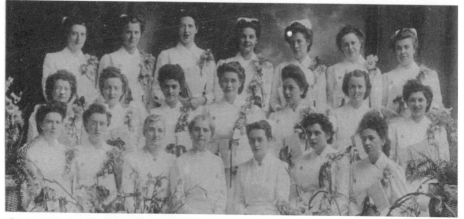

Grace Hospital School of Nursing graduating class of 1945 with three of their teachers, all of whom were Salvation Army Officers.

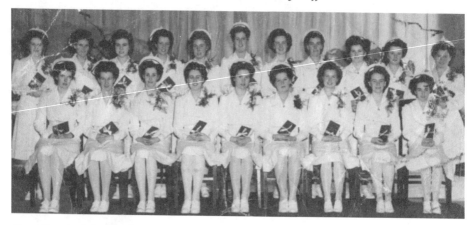

St. Clare's School of Nursing graduating class of 1947.

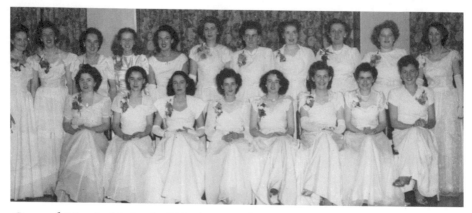

General Hospital School of Nursing graduating class of 1948.

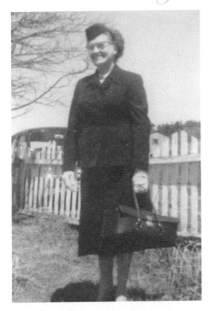

Ethel Williams in navy uniform worn by Public Health
Nurses in the winter.

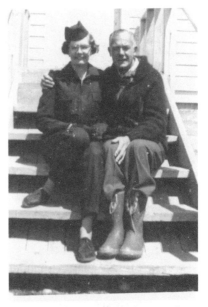

Jane Hutchings on the steps of
her clinic in Cowhead. Note her
uniform included slacks to accommodate the northern climate and
modes of transportation.

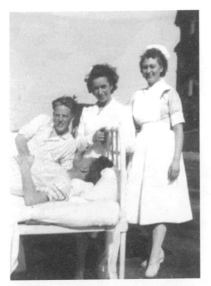

Ruby Dewling and classmate
with surgical patients. Patient
stays in hospital were often so
long that it was not unusual to
move the patients outside on
warm sunny days.

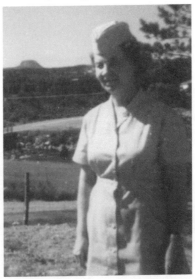

Elizabeth Avery in summer
uniform worn by Public Health
Nurses.

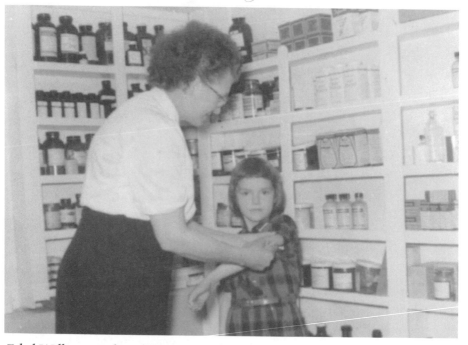

Ethel Williams in her clinic on Woody Island with the stock of supplies and medicines used by the public health nurse in rural areas.

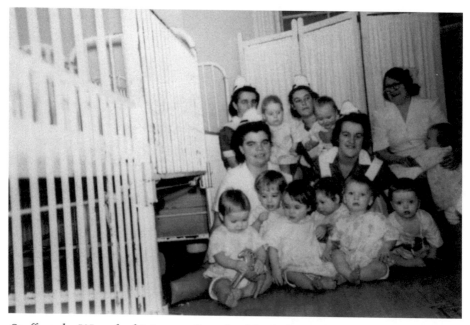

Staff at the Waterford Manor where healthy babies of unwed mothers were housed.

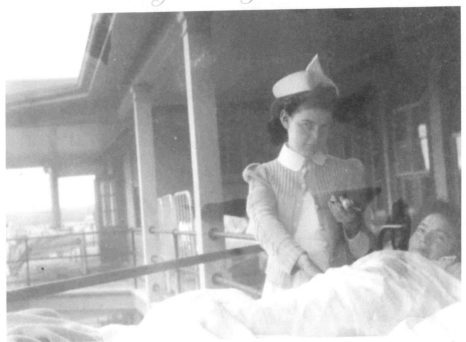

Nurse taking a patient's vital signs on the veranda of the Sanatorium. Fresh air was important for the treatment of tuberculosis.

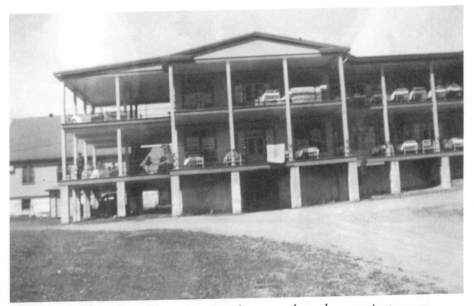

The back of the Sanatorium showing the verandas where patients were placed during the day to get fresh air.

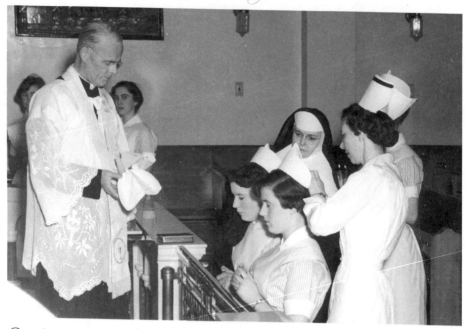

Capping ceremony taking place six months after entering St. Clare's School of Nursing; a milestone for the student nurse.

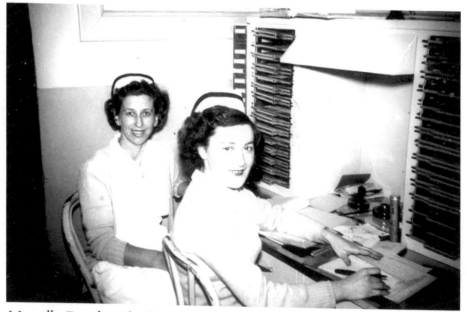

Marcella French and colleague at the nurses' station.

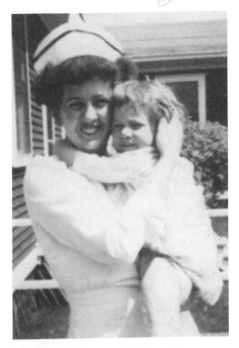

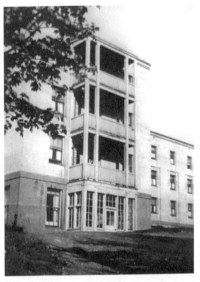

The King Edward V Residence.
Nursing students reportedly
hung their hats and gloves in
the trees when leaving for a
social evening downtown and
picked them up before returning
to the residence.

Griffen holding a child at the
Sunshine Camp, where children
went to recover from polio.

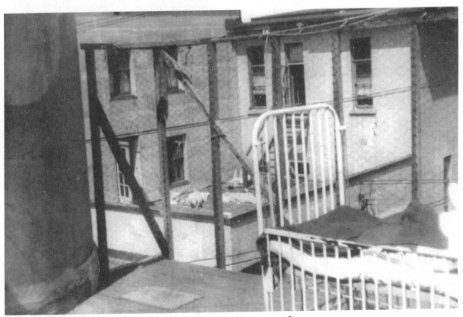

The roof where nurses would suntan on warm days.

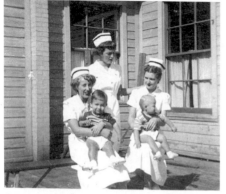

Nurses and patients at Orthopedic Hospital.

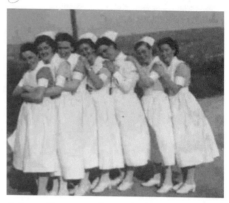

Marcella French and classmates in 1939.

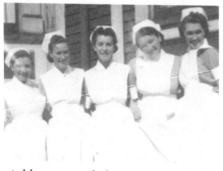

Ashbourne and classmates in 1942.

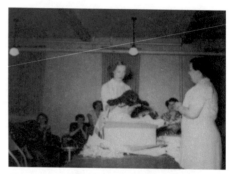

Party for Phyllis Barrett upon her resignation as Director of Nursing because of pregnancy.

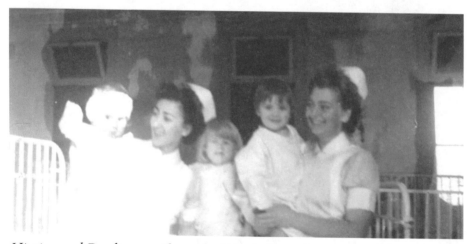

Higgins and Dewling on Alexander Ward, the pediatric unit of the General Hospital.

CHAPTER 7:
Nursing in General Hospitals

"The patient is the most important person in the hospital and they never complained about what we did to them." Story (48)

Nursing in general hospitals for these women was very similar to nursing in general hospitals today. In St. John's patients were grouped according to their health problem, e.g. medicine or surgery, or according to age, e.g. pediatrics. Nurses choosing to work in a general hospital in the city had a choice of where they worked, e.g. medicine or pediatrics. In the 1930s and 1940s, a nurse would be invited to stay on staff after graduation provided there was a vacancy. Nurses who stayed to work at the hospital where they studied had a distinct advantage over those opting to work outside the city in that they knew the rules and routines of the hospital and were prepared to handle most things they likely encountered in practice.

Nurses choosing to work in a general hospital in such areas as Twillingate, Gander and Corner Brook had to be more versatile. The wards in these agencies were smaller and often had patients with mixed health problems. Subsequently the nurses' work was more varied and often the nurse was expected to work in more than one area. For example, when on evenings the nurse might find herself leaving the ward to help deliver a baby or to assist in the operating room if there was an emergency. Clearly the expectation of nurses working in general hospitals outside St. John's was that they be multi-skilled. Nurses working in general hospitals outside St. John's worked scheduled shifts and were not constantly on call as were their colleagues in the cottage hospitals or nursing stations.

Rural General Hospitals: While many graduates chose to work in the hospital where they studied, others chose to work in general hospitals outside St. John's either to be close to family or just for the change. These hospitals functioned outside the realm of the cottage hospitals and varied in size.

They offered a wide range of services such as surgery, medicine, obstetrics and pediatrics. One such hospital was in Carbonear where Merrigan worked from 1953 to 1979; "I did maternity mostly. There were a lot of babies born there at the time [some of whom she delivered when the doctor was not present]. But mostly the doctor was there. The hospital was mainly surgery at first. Yes, it was all one place. Later they divided it up into Obstetrics and Surgical. We had really good doctors; Dr. Rowe, Dr. Drover, Dr. Wells, and Dr. Murray. They are the ones I remember."

Griffen worked in Corner Brook for six months in the late 40s prior to the opening of the new hospital, having been recruited by her friend; "I never saw such a mess in all your life! It was horrible the way it was run. And not only that, when you worked nights...now you didn't work as hard...you worked your eight hours. But if you were on the maternity part of the hospital, you had to go out and do home deliveries."

Some nurses went to Twillingate because they wanted to work with Dr. Olds. Ashbourne had not been to Twillingate before she went there to work. "It's just we thought we'd go for a change. There were all kinds of patients: obstetrics patients and...tuberculosis patients. They had a children's ward downstairs, a small one, but the others were all above. I liked it all. I liked the OR best. But when they were operating, they did deliveries on the wards. The nurses did the deliveries, whenever the doctors were operating." House, "Well see, I came back to Twillingate. I wanted to work with Dr. Olds. [He] was an American doctor who came here in 1933. At that time, the American students would come for the summer to get experience. So he came there for one year as a student and he liked Newfoundland, so he went back [to the States] and finished, he came back to Twillingate to work for one year but he was there until he died. Oh, he was a wonderful doctor! He did everything. I mean, I've known him to have an appendectomy done and get up off the table and go and see a patient. And he would give blood and they would take the blood and he would get up and give it to someone else. I mean, I think for a couple of years, he was the only doctor there. And that hospital served all of Notre Dame Bay. I worked with him from 1947 to 1951. He went everywhere by horse and sleigh. Twillingate is not that big a place but we had about ninety patients with everything. The Corner Brook doctors didn't like Dr. Olds because we had an awful lot of patients from Corner Brook that would go out there to him."

General Duty Nursing: In St. John's nurses could work on a ward or in a specialized area such as the operating room. Whiteway worked at the General Hospital on surgery for about nine years after she graduated. She did not go there immediately after graduation because there was no job available. Following a one year break she returned to Crowdy Ward as charge nurse. She worked there from 1935-46. She provides a very comprehensive picture of what nursing was like on a surgical floor in the late 1930s: "There was no nurse's aides. That came after. We had to keep the heaters clean; we had to clean out from under the heaters. I remember it (laughter). And washing all the beds. You'd give the patients water to wash in the morning. Baths were done after breakfast. You served breakfast first. Now you'd only have three or four baths a day, because most of the people there, they could wash themselves. There'd be only so many operations a week, and so they'd be getting better. And then you wouldn't have so much to do, see? Every day, nearly, there'd be somebody getting something done. You had your dressings to make then. We used to have to make all our own dressings and package them. So we didn't have very much time in between. We all worked together. I mean I'd gave baths too. I did whatever I could. After lunch. Now 2:00 p.m. to 4:00 p.m., you'd come back from lunch and you had to scrub the baths then and straighten all the beds. You had visitors from 2:00 p.m. to 4:00 p.m. Well that's the time you did whatever like you had to... clean up your bathrooms or do your linen cupboards. Write up the charts. I had to write up the charts every day. The patients didn't read them. Every morning the doctors would come. You'd have to make rounds with the doctors. We didn't stop very much. Oh yes you had to go for your evening meal. A half an hour. The nighttime routine was different. Well you didn't leave the ward in the nighttime. When you were on night duty, you were on by yourself [and] one graduate. Sometimes on nights you would have fulminations...to changes every couple of hours...it was...hot compresses. And if there was treatment or anything you had to do. Then you had to clean all the bedpans, sterilize them, and the bottles. And we had to comb all the heads (laughter). That was a job we had to do on nights. Oh yes, we're looking for nits. And there used to be lots of them in those days. An appendix was about ten days before they'd get their stitches out. And then a couple of days more and then they'd go home. Now a hernia would be about 16 days (laughter). A big change isn't it? Now they weren't allowed out of bed for 16 days. And then they'd get out and after seven days, they'd go home. That's what I can remember. But there was no such thing as getting up in the chairs and sit in bed stuff like they do now. Everything had to be kept clean. You had to clean the lockers, the beds, the floors, the bath-rooms. And you had to sterilize everything. That's the reason why I think that we got no infections. If there was an infection the nurse would have to see the matron who was very strict. And I was responsible, see because I was the one that was the one [to do the explaining]. That's the differ-ence too I think, you know, is that the nurse was responsible." In Story's description of the nurses' duties on day shift in the late 1940s and 50s the only notable difference from Whiteway's account is that nurses were no longer responsible for housekeeping duties: "At 10:00 o'clock you had your nourishment break. By then you should have had all of your patients done with the beds made and everything. Then, you would put on a clean apron and bib and continued on doing the dressings. So, while we were on coffee break the maids were sweeping and mopping the floors. We did not have to learn how to make the dressings because it was something that we saw everyday. It was all the same as a student and we would just follow through. A lot of it was routines and rituals but I guess that was the old background of the military hospitals."

Treatment modalities did not advance significantly from the 1930s to the 1940s. Tobin, "[The biggest thing you had were the dressings]. Yes and stoops. A stoop was a heavy blanket put in hot water. You had two sticks to ring it out and you would have to put that on somebody's leg, espe-cially, someone with cellulitis or something. I remember this one persons' leg was as big as my body and you had to do all of this yourself. We also had to make mustard poultices for on their chests and hot compresses." Sister Fabian, "It was amazing that with so little we had such good results. I think spirituality had a big part in it. The mothers would be there walk-ing the floor and praying. A lady came in one day with a 9 year old child from Bay Roberts and the child was blue. Apparently, Dr. Drover told her that the child would not survive the road. Anyway, when she came in, Dr. Harry Roberts was the doctor and he told her that it was too late and he thought she was going. Well, the mother knelt down on the floor and she said, 'Dear God, don't take her, she is all that I have.' And the child started to breathe. People did not depend a lot on medical care because there was not much in Newfoundland at that time, so they depended on themselves and what prayer could do for them. She had pneumonia. She seemed to do well. There were a lot of things like that happen in the earlier days."

Operating Room (OR): One of the specialty areas which seemed to attract a lot of nurses was the operating room. Bruce worked in the operating room immediately after graduation; "I loved [the operating room]. Our supervisor, Lillian Stevenson, was a tremendously knowledgeable person. She was a good teacher and I would say in my eyes, she was a marvelous nurse who really knew her work. I learned a lot from her and I remember a lot. I have already told you that my memories of my training are very pleasant but my memories of the operating room have to be the happiest ones. We used to spend some time in the Cystoscopic Room, where the cystoscopics were done. We also would look after all of the instruments, make sure everything was in order, and setting up the trays. You were the scrub nurse and you would go in and put on your gown and gloves and set up the trays for the doctor. Being an operating room nurse, you had to be one step ahead; whatever the doctor needed you wanted to have it there. The scrub nurse was also in charge of the draping of the patient and having things in order. The circulating nurse did not wear a gown and as the name implies, she circulated. If anything had to be brought in from outside you were available to tend to that. You were not scrubbed up. Then of course, when the operations for the day were over, you were in the room with the autoclave, folding the laundry and doing the autoclaving. The OR slips were typed up for the next day and the times [for surgery] and all that sort of thing was done. In the morning when we went on we brought in the necessary things on the various tables, and the float nurse and the scrub nurse then opened them. The call nurse would get things ready. Once the cases were done, if all rooms were not working at one time, there would be plenty to do. At that time there were five rooms."

Mifflin worked in the OR at the Grace which also included working in the Case Room when necessary; "I was in the operating room and that is all I ever did. Any kind of surgery would be covered in the OR. Dr. Jamieson, was the one who used to give the anesthetic; he did not always give anesthetic but mostly he did. There would only be two of us [nurses]. We had a student or two which would come up from the floors to get their training. They would help out with folding at the end of the day. We always had students. If there was an emergency it [the OR] would be open at night. I remember getting out of the bed at 3:00 o'clock in the morning and going back to the Grace for an emergency. There were a lot of times I had to go in the middle of the night when I was on call. I believe we had two days off, I am not quite sure about this but I know that we got more than the supervisors did. There would be nothing booked for Saturday or Sunday. We used the weekend to get our goods ready for the next week. We had to fold and autoclave all of our supplies. We had our own [autoclave] up in the workroom and there were two tanks for boiling water. When we would get the autoclave full we would run it, then we would fill it again when it was done. I remember one time, I was out on the road one Sunday afternoon and we had a Cesarean section on Monday morning. Grace was on for the weekend and I was not sure if she had known about the Cesarean. So I rang in to tell her because we had a special bundle for Cesareans; the hole went right down over the stomach. I wanted to make sure it was sterilized for the next day. But she had it nailed when I called, she was very good. First, when you are there, you wonder if you will live through it. But after a few weeks, you become used to it. For Cesareans we had to use those big sponges with strings on them. We would wring them out in the hot water and the doctor would do the incision. We had to make sure we had them sterilized and ready for use. Usually, after we would use them, we would sterilize them right away and they would be ready again. At first it is [scary working in the OR], but after a while it is second nature to you. In the beginning, I would go to bed at night and I would think about what was on the go for the next day and I would have all of that done before the morning came. But after a few weeks, I would not look at the board until I got in the next morning. Well, the further on you got, the more responsibility you were given. For instance, if you were on night duty, you would be on by yourself. But that too seems second nature after a while."

Although it was included as part of her OR duties, Mifflin did not enjoy the case room; "I will never forget Miss Thomas. She came to the Grace and stayed there the rest of her lifetime. She was always in charge of the case room. Anyway, operating nurses had to take turns in the case room on Sundays. This one day I told Miss Thomas that I did not mind being on duty but I did not like the responsibility because I did not like the case room very much. Well, she jumped on me; she did not like that very much. So, I took the responsibility and ended up having five deliveries from the time I went on to the time I went off. Dr. O'Regan came in one day and there were several women in labour. This one woman in particular delivered in a real hurry before he could get there. So, when he came in I told him that I had to deliver the baby and that he should have been here. He told me that he did not know when the babies were coming, only Miss Thomas knew that!"

Private Duty Nursing: Another opportunity available to St. John's nurses was private duty nursing. Initially nurses went into private duty nursing if they were between positions or wanted to only work for a short time. After marriage when they were no longer allowed to work in hospitals, many nurses chose private duty until they had children. Bruce, "I did a fair amount of private duty, meanwhile, I was having my family and at that time you were home maybe a couple of years whatever was necessary. The majority was in the hospital but I did do it on occasion in the home." Tobin opted for private duty after graduation in September 1944 because she did not want to go to work until December; "I wanted a couple of months off, but I did do a little bit of private duty at the Grace during that period. I was on with Dr. Kyle and there were no private rooms then, you only had a screen around your bed if you were a private patient." Dalley, "I did private nursing then for a while, mostly in the Grace. I knew the Grace. Well it would be like a doctor's wife or some big person like that. It wouldn't be no ordinary person."

Nurses doing private duty were independent practitioners and their salaries were paid by the patient. The amount they were paid was set by the Newfoundland Graduate Nurses Association. Dalley, "That's what they would give you...$60.00 a month. I suppose the people paid the hospital and they paid me." Bruce, "As a private duty nurse, working 12 hours, it was $5.00 a day. Psychiatry was $7.00 a day. You did not have days off because there was no one to relieve you." Nurse remembers one patient, "I did do private duty nursing. I did some nursing at St. Clare's. I do remember doing a chap from Buchans but I think that was much later when I had my family. Private duty on the third floor and the chap was from Buchans. The company there was paying me."

Private duty nurses cared for patients with all kinds of conditions, both in the hospital and/or in their home. In either setting they were responsible for all aspects of patient care. Dalley, "Mostly, it was patients that would have operations, big operations...serious operations. I remember one of them was [a doctor's] wife. She was in there but I don't remember what was wrong with her. But I do remember one thing about her – every evening at 3:00 o'clock, I'd have to make her this lemon tea! She had to have that. She was in there two weeks." Bruce outlines the nurse's duties when caring for the patient at home; "You did everything for that patient. You changed the linens, ran the baths, did the medications, did the dressings, and carried out the doctor's orders. That was usually a 12 hour duty in the hospital. You made tea and carried trays along with your nursing duties. You still did your dressings and medications and what not. Of course, this patient was not a very ill patient. It was in a home atmosphere and it was a very happy time. I remember I was in with this older lady around Christmas time. She asked me if I could play the piano. At that time, I did play. So, she asked me to play a carol for her. I remember going into the living room and playing and singing Little Town of Bethlehem for her and she was so appreciative. I found it a very rewarding experience. If they had a visitor, you would leave them for the time to have their visit. But you remained around if they needed anything." Private duty nursing was a short term option for the nurse and the work wasn't always challenging. Dalley, "I liked it but I didn't…I'd rather be in the thick of things, I tell you, in the hospital working at everything!"

Non-Nursing Duties: These nurses worked in health care in a time when there were no specialists in nursing or medicine. Subsequently both nurses and doctors performed multiple roles. In addition, there were not the categories of health care workers that exist today. This circumstance was not unique to rural hospitals. Even in St. John's hospitals, nurses were expected to carry out skills they had not been trained for in nursing school. Dalley worked for about a year in the x-ray department of the Grace Hospital; "Well I used to take x-rays and stuff. I didn't learn it but I learned it from him after I got there, a lot of it. That was Dr. William Roberts' son. He was an x-ray technologist or radiologist. I wasn't particularly keen on it, so I didn't stay there very long. I was always afraid of moving the things from one side to another…I was going to do something wrong with a machine. Well that's the way it is, I guess, in x-ray. I didn't want to do that." At St. Clare's the Sisters did further preparation before returning to the hospital to assume additional roles. Sister Fabian, "There were seven nursing Sisters at St. Clare's when we started and they were all trained in the United States. Without exception, they did extra work before they came back. When they came back they were probably involved in two or three different services. For example, Sister Magdalene was supervising Pediatrics when I was in training and she was also an x-ray technician and was in charge of x-ray. Sister Loretto was on the surgical floor but she also gave anesthetics and she supervised the operating room."

Dewling worked in the lab at the General Hospital but was required to do a course in preparation, "Dr. Joseph always had a nurse in charge of the lab at the General. [He] was Chief of Medicine. One day I was so upset with the way that they treated me in emergency, I was talking to a nurse in the outpatients getting ready to go to lunch. Well, one of the nursing supervisors came over and caught me washing my hands in the sink; she grabbed me by the collar and told me that that was not my sink and I could not wash my hands there. I was so upset by this and I could not stand it any more because there were several other incidents like that one. So when I walked out in the corridor I ran into Dr. Josephsen who looked at me and told me that I looked mad enough to do anything and asked me if I would transfer to the lab. So, then I went and did a lab course and worked with Dr. Josephsen. I took all of the bloods in the hospital, I did gastric analysis, I did all of the chemistry, hematology, and pathology; I did everything. Also, Dr. Josephsen used to have me read slides and stand over my shoulder while I read them. I stayed there until I went to the University of Toronto."

Administration: Nurses who assumed supervisory or administrative positions in a general hospital rarely had formal preparation but generally received on the job training for the role and responsibilities. The duties of the supervisor varied depending on the agency, the department or the shift she worked. On days, each ward had its own supervisor, or Head Nurse as she was called.

Story began her administrative career as a Head Nurse on a medical ward. When asked how she learned the role of Head Nurse she responded, "You sort of picked it up as you went along. The Head Nurse had to fill out the time sheets, pick up reports, arrange lunch hours and nourishment breaks [for staff]. Students were the staff...I spent half my days looking after patients although I was the supervisor because we were so short staffed." On evenings and nights, she was called the evening or night supervisor and assumed responsibility for the entire hospital. Sister Fabian, "I was supervisor for six months of night duty and I worked in the case room. We did a lot of things then that you cannot do today. When I was in charge of Pediatrics I was supervising and I was teaching it and I was also in charge of emergency. But emergency then was nothing compared to now; you would probably have two or three patients a day and they were small things because the General Hospital was getting all of the heavier work, naturally." When she left the nursing department to move into hospital administration, Sister Fabian had the responsibility of determining staff quotas on the various units of St. Clare's; "When I came back from Toronto and worked in Pediatrics, Pediatrics was at the end of the stick and there was not enough staff. So, when I went into administration, I was accused of being partial to Pediatrics and giving them more staff than they should have. But they don't realize children need more staff to care for them. I don't think that I was partial to it but maybe I was; if they asked for more staff I probably gave it to them." Avery, "I came back to Newfoundland and I worked at the Grace in the case room...a full year of nights in the case room. The only break I had from it was when Miss Benson and Miss Morgan took their holidays together and I was left in charge. I was the night supervisor of the hospital for a month. I would have to go down and check the reports in all of the places to see who was sick and who wasn't and ask about all of the patients. If anyone was sick, I would pop into their room and see if there was anything wrong. If there were any complaints they would come to me and I would have to get in contact with the doctor. Also, I would have to write a report during the night to pass to the day supervisors. Pretty much, I was keeping an eye on everything and making sure nothing went astray. [As night supervisor I was not responsible for staffing] that would have been done in the after-noon. Somebody might ring in but the day staff would be responsible to find a nurse for the rest of the day." Bruce, who was night supervisor at the General Hospital, tells a similar story about her duties which she shared with another supervisor: "You went on in the afternoon and after hearing the report, you made the rounds over the entire hospital. By the time you have made complete rounds, you knew exactly where the seri-ously ill patients were located. These were the places that you gave more attention to and concentrated on. You made general rounds again before you came off in the morning and you would then write your report. You had to know who was seriously ill. There were two supervisors. They were senior students, sometimes you would find a graduate. There was a doc-tor's area in the main building. Doctor's were always available."

When Barrett was offered the position of Director of Nursing at the General Hospital in 1951, she saw an opportunity to make changes in the nursing department, "So I thought about it...and I said now, this is my opportunity to get the General assessed. So he [Dr. Miller] asked me who I'd like to do it and I told him I'd like for Gladys Sharpe – she was my teacher at the U of T (University of Toronto) and she was Director of Nursing at the Toronto Western and they had put in all new ideas. And he got back to me and told me 'Yes, she could come.' That was it. The General was a mess. I phoned her. She was surprised. And she got back to me and said, 'Yes' she'd come. I explained to her what I wanted. Anyway, she came. And she interviewed all the Head Nurses and Supervisors. And we met her and had a reception. Dr. Miller and the Minister of Health, Dr. Chalker, were all there. And anyway, she went in and she had a free hand in everything. And she assessed the whole...interviewed everybody and asked them all what she wanted to do. She was there more than a week and then she interviewed me and asked me how I felt. And I said, 'Well, I felt all right.' And I said to her, 'Now don't feel you have to recommend me. Recommend me if you feel I can do the job.' So she recommended me but she wanted me to go and spend some time with Edith Young who was the Director of Nursing at the Ottawa Civic. So I went there. They sent me. I suppose I must have been there a couple of weeks. And I did all the shifts there; day, evening and night – did it all. And came back and went into the General. The first thing that I did, according to Edith Young, the left hand didn't know what the right hand was doing all over the place, so we got policy books. And everything went out under my name as the Director and everything that was changed, it went out in a policy. And how we developed them was we had a little morning conference of the head nurses, every morning, for about five minutes. Well, five or six minutes. But not long because I couldn't leave. And everything developed out of that. So then we put in the eight hour shift. But they only had a day off a week. You 7:00 a.m. to 7:00 p.m. and a day off. And then, when the budget came down, we had something like over a 100 extra staff graduates. And we put it in right away. And then I wanted a permanent person for evenings and a permanent person for nights. They were called Assistant Directors. Then we had a person that we could move when they had their day off. So we were covered – fully. For seven days a week. So anyway then I started in and sent people away and Pauline Rowe went to the Harper, in Detroit. Mary Feehan went to the Toronto Western. Gert Tobin went to the Toronto Western. Steve went away...Stevenson in the OR. I would write the Director, send a tentative program. They would just take them and give them all the experience in different areas that they wanted. And it worked like a charm! And then, the nursing assistants. The nursing assistants then had no program only...scattered. So then we developed a program. Nine months and then three months of experience. And then they had a little graduation. And that was the first class of trained or educated nursing assistants." When asked if the other hospitals were aware of what was happening at the General, Barrett responded, "We didn't co-operate then like they do now, but they knew. Hannah Janes, Colonel, was at the Grace. I believe it was Sister Fabian [at St. Clare's]. And I'd call them and meet with them and tell them...and then they started to institute certain things."

In 1963, Story moved up to the Director of Nursing at the General, a position she held until her retirement in 1983: "Initially, I started off trying to educate people; so we would have head nurse and supervisor meetings about improvements that could have been made. At least I had the opportunity to give my input. We were in charge of the school and the nursing service and we only had two associates. Again, a lot of the agonies were on staffing because there were not enough nurses...we set up all the policies and practices. There were not too many formal contacts through the departments. Also, there are so many things that you don't have to teach because they would learn it from experiences that other people would have had. There was one continuous effort to improve around 1966 or 1967 because there were federal consultants set up in nursing to do activity studies. At that time, health care costs were going up. You were looking at everyone else, seeing how you could do it cheaper and the only way you could save money was to cut staff. So, we had these studies done to see if the nurses were doing their work and that went on for about three or four years. So, there was one continuous effort to try and improve patient care and practice. Then we got in the business of medical school and teaching hospital. We spent a lot of time planning a new hospital including, structures and setting up an organization. That went on for 10 years almost. I think with all of these activity studies, the other departments began to feel that they were there to accommodate whatever the nurses were doing."

Teaching: The three hospitals in St. John's each had a nursing school and relied heavily on the students to staff the hospital. In fact the number of students admitted to the program generally corresponded to the need for staff in the hospital. Story, "It [class size] varied until they opened the new wing with the extra beds. Classes started increasing when the beds did." Even with the increase, class size was still small compared to today. Roche, "...[Classes] would not be that large in comparison to some of them today; there were probably about 30 students in each." There were nursing teachers, however, they were usually responsible for large numbers of students and several wards. Subsequently the clinical supervision of students usually fell to the nursing supervisor and ward staff. Story, "As a clinical supervisor I had more than one ward, so I had several head nurses working underneath me. We had the entire class to be responsible for. Some of them would be on the medical floor and others would be all over the building. I was only in this clinical thing for a year and then the next year I went off to Toronto. I worked in surgery and medicine then. We learned some things from Toronto. We tried to get some coordination between what the students were learning and what they were doing. Then, Phil Barrett got busy trying to change the nursing program. The nursing students were the staff. We tried to have more classes but it was difficult because they were also the nursing staff."

In the mid 1950s the structure of the nursing program was changed and the two plus one program was introduced. It was at this point that the hospital's reliance on students was reduced somewhat. At that time, the nurse intern year was introduced and the school of nursing took complete control of the students in first and second year. While these program changes took students out of the control of service it also left a gap in available staff. So about the same time measures were implemented to replace them on the wards and a program introduced to train the nursing assistants. Story, "That is when they were doing the preliminary work on getting nursing assistants trained, which happened in 1955. They needed this done to replace the nursing students who went out."

By the late 1960s and early 1970s the schools of nursing were attracting nursing staff from service to teach in the school. Oakley, "My husband died in November of 1966 and they asked me to go back as an instructor at the Grace for first and third year maternity students. So, I went back for nine years and worked until I was nearly 70 years old. That was from 1967 to 1976. There was a lot of differences. When I was an instructor, I was only on the floor...they had the nurses teaching them." When she trained her teachers were doctors, except for Miss Thomas. Barron was also seconded from nursing service in the early 1970s to teach in the school of nursing: "Because now they needed someone in nursing education, and they always needed somebody with med-surg and they were always sending someone over to talk to me, you know... you'd be good at this, and you could do this and you can do that, and I didn't want it. I felt that if I wanted to be an instructor, I was knowledgeable and I did know my med-surg material well, and they used to send me students over with the patients...I did clinical on med-surg for first year. And after that I went into the classroom." Barron taught for 14 years. "For the first seven I taught first years and second years in the classroom...and for the next seven, I coordinated the intern year. Like I put a lot of emphasis on different things, you know, even on their deportment, how they dressed, how clean they looked, their dress, even their shoes. I mean...there was no way they'd passed me by with dirty shoes."

From their inception, each of the schools of nursing was directly linked to the hospital and was under the direction of the nurse in charge in the hospital. It was not until the mid 1970s that steps were taken to change that structure and make the school of nursing independent of nursing service. Nicolle (47), "The only time I could really make the decisions...we had committees then see, the only time was after Jan [Story] came there...I took it over then. I took it over hook, line and sinker. And after a while I got to become Director of the school." Despite all the efforts to make the school independent of nursing service and not to use students for staffing, it was not until the 1980s that hospitals stopped using students to relieve staff particularly at vacation times. Nicolle, "I told [one of the Directors at another school] our first and second year students are going until New Year's. They're going to have a Christmas vacation. Before that the students were relieving [staff] at Christmas."

Salaries: The 1930s was the era of the Depression. Nurses were among a small number of women who received an independent salary. French recalls, "I know my first check was for $54.00. Whiteway reports, "Salary at that time was "$53.00 a month." This would be a reasonable salary for the time. Sister Fabian, who as a nun worked at St. Clare's Hospital, a private institution, "Money didn't really mean that much to us; if we got it we got it but if we didn't, it wasn't personal." When asked about salary, Bruce who worked as an OR nurse, responded "...I can't be too accurate, but it was less than $100.00. But you must remember...we lived in residence. We had our meals and a beautiful room and your laundry."

After the war was over Newfoundland was still in a rather desperate financial situation so salaries did not rise dramatically. In 1947, Penney worked at the Fever; "We started at $80.00 a month. That was big money then. There wasn't a lot of people making $80.00 a month." Story recalled her salary at the beginning of her career along with the additional benefits which increased its value. "I think we got $90.00 per month. But then, we had all of our uniforms supplied, we lived in residence, and we were deducted $11.00 a month for our meals. Our laundry was taken care of as well. It was like being at home. There was one nurse that never went out; she never had to and with helping yourself to the supplies on the ward, you never had to buy yourself a Band-Aid. There were some that never bought a pill." Dewling also lived in residence, as did all single women, but they were no longer under the control of the house mother. Dewling recalls, "I lived in residence until I got married. It did not cost me anything. But we did not get paid very much. After you graduated, you were on your own; you were not subject to all of the rules and regulations. There were two of us in adjoining rooms with a little sitting room and a kitchen out around the corner if we wanted to cook our own meals. We could not afford to live out with the salary that we got." Roche received a higher salary because she was teaching. "In 1949 when I started, I think my salary was $88.00 per month. I don't remember. But I think when I was teaching, I got about $20.00 more per month. We did not have the graduated salary scales that they have today. They only came in over the last 20 years or so."

Through the 1950s and 60s women were paid less than men in all occupations and nurses were not unionized. By the 1970s, Williams reports, "Before I left Woody Island and came over here, I was only paid $450.00 a month." Even by the early 80s, salaries had not risen dramatically in terms of today's salaries but from Avery's recollections her salary had increased 500 or 600 percent over the course of her career. "As a registered nurse, my first paycheck was less than $100.00 for a month. I finished in August and I did not go home for a few months. While I was in Old Perlican Hospital, the Government paid me. It went up very gradually; I got a bit more when I was on the mainland. I might have gotten $500 .00 or $600.00 by the time I retired in 1982." Indeed most nurses felt that they derived more benefit from their profession than mere money and although these were strong women they did not feel it was right to ask for more.

CHAPTER 8:
Other Agencies Employing Nurses

"I sort of suited The Waterford and I really liked it." Strong (37)

"It was a very interesting and rewarding hospital (Merchant Navy Hospital) in which to work." St. George (42)

Many of the agencies where these nurses worked no longer exist. For some they no longer served a purpose, while for others the services were incorporated into general hospital services. In all cases the existence of these agencies reflected the times, the rampant communicable diseases and the large military presence because of the war and socioeconomic conditions. All these agencies with the exception of the Gander Airport were housed in St. John's and acted as referral centers for the whole province. Nursing skills were needed for a wide variety of institutions and agencies, as they are today. In the past, the two major specialty hospitals were the Hospital for Mental and Nervous Diseases, known as the Waterford Hospital today, and the Sanatorium, where patients with tuberculosis were housed and treated. Other agencies where nurses were employed were the Infirmary (Poor House), Fever, Merchant Navy and Orthopedic Hospitals. The Public Health Department ran an agency on Waterford Bridge Road where babies of unwed mothers were housed until adopted, and in keeping with the lack of a road system in Newfoundland Public Health also used ships such as the *Christmas Seal* and the *Lady Anderson*, which travelled around Newfoundland bringing health care to outport communities. In addition to being places of employment, the Sanatorium, Waterford, and the Fever were agencies where students affiliated as part of their nursing program.

The Sanatorium: 'The San' was located on the outskirts of St. John's and functioned as the provincial treatment center for patients with pulmonary tuberculosis. All nursing students were rotated through the center once affiliations were introduced. As well, there were nurses on permanent staff. St. George, "Following graduation I accepted a position at the St. John's Sanatorium on Topsail Road. The nurse's duty was to make a round when you came on duty to see how your patients were doing. The nurse's aides made the beds." Nurse describes her duties as a student there, "We had to put dust bane on the floors and sweep it and we had to open every window and the patients all had mitts and sweaters and…because the idea was fresh air." French worked at the Sanatorium most of her working life. She describes the layout of the hospital: "There were wards and the males and females were separated with the females on wards 7 and 8, and the males on wards 1 and 2. Then we had the south wing, where they did some minor surgery. Finally, they brought in pre-teenagers and eventually they had the children's ward. I worked on the men's ward mostly and we had about twenty odd. Then they had the exercise patients out on the veranda. Yes, and it was cold out there. We used to have to wear gloves and sweaters to make the beds out there. At that time, we had a building called the Hut, that was used for everything; church on Sunday, concerts on Monday's, whichever. Then, there was what we called the south wing, which was made up of sicker patients. Therefore, when they did surgery, all patients would end up in the south wing. You see, they did the surgery down at the General. They would go down to the General and have their surgery and stay down there for a couple of weeks. But eventually, they opened up an operating room in the Sanatorium."

Treatment for tuberculosis changed over time. At the beginning there was very little hope for a patient who contracted the disease. French, "Before they got the Tb drugs it was purely rest and food…yes, in the beginning because there was no drugs. But when they got the Tb drugs it was a godsend." St. George, "Most of the patients had complete rest for two hours in the mornings and afternoons with all the windows open for fresh air."

French, "One thing that I did not agree with was the rest period from 9:00 a.m. until 11:30 a.m. and again in the evening from 2:00 p.m. to 4:00 p.m. That was complete rest, there was no reading or anything. One day I was cleaning the veranda and came across a book, so, I asked the patient [Jerry] what the book was doing there, and he replied that he was wondering the same thing himself. Imagine making you lay down for two hours and look at the ceiling!" French also described the common treatments at the Sanatorium while she was a nurse there. One was the Pneumothorax, a treatment that was given one to three times a week and consisted of putting a needle between the ribs and injecting air into the pleural cavity. This collapsed the lung and healing could occur while the lung was at rest. Another, the Phrenic Crush was done if the cavity caused by the tuberculosis was in the base of the lung. The phrenic nerve was crushed and this would cause the diaphragm to collapse and push upward. The chest cavity would be smaller and easier to fill with air. The third and most invasive treatment was the Thorocoplasty which was performed in the OR. An incision was made in the patient's side and two or three ribs would be removed. The chest was would then fall and collapse the lung permanently. St. George, "Artificial pneumothorax and thoracoplasty were done to patients who would benefit from it weekly by Dr. D. R. Bennett, the Medical Director. Miss Ethel Wells, Registered Nurse (RN) was the Matron and Miss M. Chard, Assistant."

As patients recuperated, they progressed to the veranda outdoors and eventually they were allowed to have an exercise period. French, "Before the Tb drugs they would be in anywhere from one year to three years. When they would finally progress they would be allowed to do a half an hour of exercise. They would go out after rest period and go for a walk outdoors. They could go wherever they like for the hour that they were out. This lad came in from the army and really liked his drink. So, this day, he was on exercise and I got this phone call questioning if I had this young lad as my patient. Apparently, it was the police station and he was down at the station after going out and having a few drinks." Nurse worked at the Sanatorium for two years after the Tb drugs had been introduced. "But then when I went back on the staff, much later, there was the PAS, the INAH, the miracle drugs…and so we had tins of pills that were being given. I can't remember the blood tests but we'd routinely do that; they all had to have that, the patients. So that's what you were busy doing and they had to be weighed and bathed and, of course, then back up to the cold…not the cold area in the 50s this time, because there was quite a difference."

Because many patients stayed at the Sanatorium for long periods, they came to know each other and staff quite well and weren't above playing jokes on each other and on staff, particularly students. French, "When they were doing the surgery in the Sanatorium, even for a phrenic crush they would give you an anaesthetic. So, this one chap had a general anaesthetic and came back to his own bed, which was on the ward. It was either before Christmas or after Christmas, either way the decorations were still up. I had to check on him, so I went down during the afternoon and he was sound asleep. Apparently, someone was after picking a wreath off the wall and put it on his head and there he was, out like a light, with a Christmas wreath on his head!" Griffen worked at the Sanatorium for six months as a student, "But they were all happy in the San, I mean some of them were there two years but they sort of accepted it. I was frightened to death of tuberculosis. I was afraid of everything (laughter)! I remember one, they never did it to me but they'd probably take you, if they knew you were scared of Tb, and put you in the bed with one [of the patients]. Because they were all up to just...plain fun. Dr. Brownrigg used to do lung surgery, in those days. Then they'd be in bed but, otherwise, they were up. They could get up around all day."

The nurses became quite fond of the patients, especially the children. French, "We had a young fellow on the ward and at that stage, there was a program on one of the radio stations that would be broadcast at suppertime when the news would come on. Anyway, the little fellow had red hair and the boys used to call him the Old Red Rooster. Well, it was his birthday, so we got a gift for him and put it in a locker and somebody put it on the air on this show. They wished him a Happy Birthday and they told him to look in the Old Red Rooster's locker and there would be a present for him...then the Rotarian's were very good. We had a group that would come in and bring entertainment. Two people would have to stay on and go down with the patients when something was on the go. They would bring in singing and maybe a little play."

Once the tuberculosis drugs were introduced the incidence of Tb dropped and the Sanatorium closed. French, "I then worked at St. Clare's and retired when I was 65 years old. All of the Tb was finished and the few patients that were left were sent to Corner Brook, because there was a Sanatorium out there. But there was not very many Tb patients, just emphysema and different chronic chest diseases. So they left and that gave us 20 beds on medicine at St. Clare's and that is where we went. They also, brought the patients back for re-checks at the x-ray room in the basement. They would only come in by day. They would not stay overnight. I suppose every three to six months."

Hospital for Mental and Nervous Diseases (now the Waterford Hospital): The Mental became familiar to nurses because the nursing school affiliations required that all nursing students have a rotation there. Some returned to work there for many years. Strong worked in psychiatric nursing for most of her career: "I was a Staff Nurse from 1938 to1942 and then I was Director of Nurses from 1942 to 1949. I sort of suited the Waterford and I really liked it. It so happened that Dr. Grieves asked Miss Taylor if she had anyone she could recommend to be sent away. So, I took a course from 1937 to 1938 at Toronto Psychiatric Hospital. At that time, the only treatment they used were continuous water baths, which were very good...[and] patients worked in the laundry and in the kitchen." Patients did the work under the attendance of the housekeeping staff. [This served as an alternate patient therapy]. But a doctor in Saint John, New Brunswick had started hypoglycemic therapy and Dr. Grieves, who was the superintendent of the hospital, had gone to see the results. Following his visit, she travelled to New Brunswick to take a course in Insulin therapy. "In May of 1938, we started it in St. John's and we had great success. They stopped it because I suppose, there was never enough staff to continue and the circumstances changed in there because there was a period when there was no doctor. We had to watch them very carefully. There would be more staff on the insulin ward than on other wards. They had high doses because the aim was for them to have a coma. They would be given the high dose in the morning and they had to be watched carefully. Sometimes, they would have a convulsion. One lady came in who was suffering from deep depression. She was very poor and poorly dressed and she was pregnant. Anyway, Dr. Grieves thought 'Lets do something for her.' Well, she had a convulsion on a very low dose of insulin and she recovered perfectly. Ten years later, insulin therapy was still a primary treatment in psychiatry." King, "Insulin therapy was used very extensively in those days along with Electric Shock Treatment (ECT). We had about six patients and some of them were out-patients. They would come in to see us in the morning and we would give them a dosage of insulin that was much higher than you would take with diabetes, to the point where you would put them into several stages of coma. They would reach the coma eventually and we would terminate that by giving them glucose intravenously and this would bring the patient back to normal. The patient then would spend the rest of the day in psychotherapy or being active. [A coma] was supposed to disintegrate their psychotic thoughts. When I think back to that, it was very serious. We did have a graduate nurse that was in charge all of the time; I only worked there a very short while. On occasion, we would have a patient who would have an ECT, often called shock treatment, and they would sometimes have both of these. This was very serious; the doctor would never leave the unit during that time. If I were not in charge that day, I would be helping the nurse who gave the insulin herself. But if I happened to be in charge I would inject the insulin. I am not sure if I gave insulin because that was a very big responsibility...in the early days, there were very few drugs given. Although still, there are drugs given today that were used then. When I first saw an ECT given, the patient's head was shaved right around the temporal area and that is where the electrode was placed. We would stand and hold the padded patient because of that Grand Mal seizure that they were having. Today, they do that treatment up in recovery and they have an injection of an anti-convulsive drug and you hardly see them moving on the table. Also, there was no anesthetic; it was years later before the anesthetist came."

"In 1942, the matron was leaving and I [Strong] applied for the job but they automatically thought that Miss Callahan would fill the job. I knew nothing about administration but I did get the job with help from Dr. Grieves. Now, I was in charge of nursing assistants, graduate nurses, and later more. Some time later, Dr. Crummy had left and Dr. Grieves got sick and here I was with no doctor. Dr. Kane and Dr. McNamara would come but they had no psychiatric experience; I had to rely on someone who did. That meant I had the male side, the female side, the laundry, the kitchen, and my own duties to worry about. Dr. Grieves wanted to keep in touch. So, I used to try and keep him up to date by going out to his house on Water Street with some folders. But I was wanted everywhere and it was a pleasure to go out but it was just too much time. After a while, Dr. Grieves died and Dr. Simpson from the Naval Base used to come in and that was before there was electric treatment. I remember once there was a woman that they didn't think was going to recover from the deep depression she was in. Apparently, she did end up dying and Dr. Simpson cried when I told him. He was really upset because he knew that she was a mother. The responsibility was something terrible. It so happened that a board of local judges and lawyers used to come in and that is how we got people discharged. I would do a report on the patient, how they were doing and they [the board] would decide if she would be well enough to go home. I can't ever remember doing it out for a man. I don't know who took care of them being discharged."

Strong, "The staff had really long hours. I was at the Waterford when we started 8-hour shifts. That is when we started the rotation. There would be a shift from 8:00 a.m. to 4:00 p.m. and then another one with less staff at 4:00 p.m. to 12:00 a.m. With this system nurses knew what shift they would be on a month in advance. There was usually one or two [Registered Nurses] on nights. Really, you would have to take your hat off to the nursing assistants. They worked really hard and did everything. One morning they came and told me that a woman had hung herself in the bathroom. At that time, there was not one graduate nurse on and the poor nursing assistants were trying to cope with this; they were very tender women." King also recalls the staffing at the hospital, "Every unit had [a graduate]. Then, they had experienced nursing assistants who were a great help but they could not give medications or IVs. We also had a sick unit for anyone who needed that care. All wards were locked at that time and we were very surprised when, in later years they unlocked them. We had people who had courses and that. They came in to the Waterford to be Occupational Therapy Aides. They had skills and they knew how to do all of the knitting and sewing and they taught the patients how to do that. We had basketball and dances. The Rotary was very involved at the Waterford." As at the Sanatorium, the staff also returned to the wards during their time off to help out by taking the patients to the entertainment. King, "Yes. I think they expected us to do that but we did not mind because we enjoyed doing it. In those days, you knew everybody and you were very close."

The nurses who worked at the Waterford truly appreciated the work of the untrained nursing assistants many of whom often worked at the institution for years. These men and women, started working with the mentally ill without formal training and for many years made up the majority of the staff. King, "They were called attendants and nursing aides but we changed that. In those days when I first went there, the men were in uniforms with brass buttons. I thought that was terrible. We got them out of those uniforms and into white uniforms. They were just serge uniforms with brass buttons. It almost looked like a penitentiary type uniform. They were like guards and the patients called them guards as well. They would not hurt anyone in any way; they were very nice people." Strong, "When my children were in school all day I went back to work. I asked if I could look after the nursing assistants because I had such a warm spot in my heart for them and I thought I would like to have a hand in their education. So, I was on the teaching staff from 1960 to 1966. After that I worked with affiliating nurses." King also taught the nursing assistants: "Then, the nursing assistants had to be taught. They would do basic nursing, such as bed baths, temperatures, bed making, and interpersonal relationships. Then, at the end of their 6 month course they had a graduation ceremony apart from the student nurses. I wrote all of their names in script on their certificates but my name was not on them; that would be the director of nursing."

Some of the treatments employed at the time are still used today and some have been replaced with new and more effective therapy. Strong, "Back before there was Penicillin, they used to treat patients in the last stages of Syphilis in a fever machine. The machine would get up to very high temperatures and kill the bacteria." King worked as a manager in this unit after she returned from completing a psychiatric nursing course at McGill University. "I came right back to the Waterford Hospital. I did not actually work on the floors as a nurse because I was in the specialty areas. I worked in the fever therapy treatment for GPI [condition of the brain] and we had to give artificial fever therapy by putting the patient in the cabinet and raising their temperature to 104°. I remember it was a lot of responsibility...that was the treatment then. This was a therapy to kill bacteria. But it was not only one treatment. This would go on for a long, long time." In 1949, Strong was traveling back to Newfoundland from a visit to hospitals in the United States and Canada. Dr. Grieves had heard about a new Malaria treatment for end stage of Syphilis – patients were given a course of Malaria which ended with Quinine. He asked her to stop off in New Brunswick and see what they were doing. At his request she carried back Malarial blood, taped to her ribs, from New Brunswick to St. John's. It took her three days to get home by boat and train.

Higgins left the General Hospital to work in the operating room at the Waterford: "I had a friend in there, one of my classmates, and I decided to make a change. Dr. Brownrigg was going to do prefrontal lobotomies in there, and that interested me so I was attached to the OR and worked pre-operatively and post-operatively with the prefrontal lobotomy patients. I scrubbed for the first lobotomy that was done in Newfoundland and...I was scrubbed for five and a half hours...without a break. But I had scrubbed for Dr. Brownrigg and had scrubbed for some major surgery. It was really exciting, yes, because you did the history and, you saw the patient progress, or regress, as would be. Well, patients who were advanced in their psychosis, and were making little progress. It was the advanced patient that he did that would show more improvement... well, some were successful. I don't recall now, how many. He didn't do a lot because that took time to study that patient...how it was for two or three months. But it was an experience. I was at the Waterford only one year." King also attended this surgery: "I was in there when they did the prefrontal lobotomy. Now, students did not see that done but they saw patients post-operatively. These are long-term chronic Schizophrenic patients who are more than likely Obsessive-Compulsive who had this operation performed. The Waterford had an operating room at that time and Dr. Brownrigg did that surgery. After the surgery, the patient would have to be taught again; this would be done one on one and many of these were successful but many were not."

In addition to the medical therapies, the Waterford staff explored other therapeutic avenues for the patients. In 1949, when Newfoundland was still a country, Strong traveled to the United States and Canada to investigate the latest therapies for mental illness. "I went to the Institute for Living in Hartford Connecticut and that was very high class. I think Dr. Roberts arranged that; he thought it would be good for me to see it. When I came back from there, I arranged for us to have colored uniforms at the Waterford; I thought it would make for a better atmosphere. On my way back from Hartford, I stopped in Ontario and saw the hospitals, just to see what could be done."

The Fever: Before immunizations were used to any great extent, communicable diseases were rampant throughout the province. The Fever was a hospital, located near the General on Forest Road, where patients with these infections were sent. Godden worked at the Fever as an untrained nursing aide before going into nursing school: "Yes I worked at the Fever Hospital for years...not as a trained nurse...just went in, fresh. And worked in there for years...three years I think it was." According to Godden, the conditions prevalent at the Fever in the 1930s included, "...all kinds of conditions – Typhoid, Erysipelas, Diphtheria, Whooping Cough, Measles – all those things." Almost twenty years later the conditions treated at the Fever had not changed dramatically. Woodland, "At the Fever, [you'd have] complications of Measles which would be Pneumonia, and you'd have Tb Meningitis...and Polio. I liked it except...you had to scrub so much and my poor arms and hands were...raw! And the one in charge was very, very strict. We had to do six weeks down there. We were glad to leave there." In addition to caring for inpatients, staff at the Fever were called out when there was a suspected communicable disease. Dewling, "Anyway, we got a call one morning that there was a French fishing trawler in and some of the crew had mumps with complications. We used to do ambulance calls at the Fever. But we were dressed up pretty with a long white gown and a blue cape and off we went with the drivers. We looked after the patients coming back. Anyway, when they told me that they wanted me to attend that day, I told her that I could not speak French. She said, 'You don't have to speak French. There will be an interpreter there.' So, off I went out in the harbour aboard this trawler and I am sitting there with all of these men around me wanting me to see their Mumps. The driver was sitting beside me and I warned him not to move one inch away from me because I was so terrified and the smell on board was making me sick. I asked who could speak English and nobody could and I had to fill out this big long form. Anyway, they eventually brought an interpreter on board from Customs and he had a great kick out of the questions that I had to ask these men. Finally, we got it all filled out and I went back to the Fever with the two men and put them in bed. [They would have stayed in the hospital]...a couple of weeks and I don't know where they would have gone then." Penney also worked at the Fever for two years after graduation. She lived in residence and worked seven days a week.

St. John Ambulance: Story resigned from teaching and worked for St. John Ambulance for a couple of years: "I was teaching first aid and home nursing." This was a newly created position and she was responsible for getting St. John Ambulance moving in the province. Story, "I was there for a couple of years and then I got tired of that and went back to the General Hospital as supervisor."

The Infirmary: Merrigan worked at the Infirmary in the west end of the city near Victoria Park for a number of years before she got married in 1948. Merrigan, "I also worked at the Infirmary in St. John's, people used to call that the Poor House. Some people would never think of calling it the Poor House, I never did. I suppose it was because people were poor when they went there. But I liked it there. It was just for people who could not get around. Something like a nursing home. In the hospital at the Infirmary, we would wash them and get the trays ready. Miss Vey was in charge there at one time before I left. It was clean." Merrigan estimated that the number of patients was about 80 at any one time. Most needed some degree of nursing care, "We did eight hour shifts there...we would work every day. There was quite a few [nurses]; I think there was two floors in the Infirmary."

Waterford Manor: Puddister worked at the home for seven months before getting married: "I nursed with Public Health on Waterford Bridge

Road when I graduated. It was in a house, which is now a bed and break-fast. I worked just with children there...only babies. About thirty. Just looking after so many babies each day. [She reported to] the nurse. Her name was Miss Casey. The other one was from England."

Industrial Nursing (Dosco): Moakler, "I worked with Dosco as an indus-trial nurse...five years...'52 to '57...there was the mines there and we had to go to work in the mine; there was an office upstairs, the nursing office, and we'd just sit there and wait to see if there was any accidents...and we were there just in case there was accidents. It was like a little hospital room. And we had to be around the clock, of course, so we did shift work but when you were on in the evenings, you could lie down; there was a cot there and you could lie down. [There were four nurses]."

Merchant Navy Hospital: St. George, "In 1946 I accepted a position at the Merchant Navy Hospital on Water Street West. It was a beautiful old family residence with three floors, the nurse's residence on the third floor. The first and second floors were for patients, x-ray room, laboratory and a treatment room where patients received quartz lamp, heating pads and physiotherapy. The patients were Portuguese, Spanish, and French sea-men. It also housed World War I and II war veterans who came for check-ups with regard to their pensions. We had an officer's ward on the second floor with five beds. When the ships came into port, the ship's agent would go on board and take the sick sailors to the hospital, accompanied by the ship's doctor and an interpreter. Dr. [Dinty] Moores was the doc-tor in charge of the Merchant Navy Hospital and Dr. J. J. Kennedy was Assistant. They would be informed [when the patient came in] and would come right away to give their diagnosis and prescribe treatment."

St. George, "In July 1948 I was offered a position as assistant x-ray tech-nician [at the hospital] and completed a course in Modern Radiographic Procedure given by General Electric Medical Products Company and the General Hospital. Dr. Bliss Murphy was with the RCAF (Royal Canadian Air Force) in Gander and he alternated with Dr. W. J. Higgins weekly to do Gastric Series Barium Enemas and to read the x-rays taken the previ-ous week. We also developed our own x-rays. When the Radiologist came for the readings, I also took the dictation. One evening I got a call back to the x-ray as a sailor had fallen in the hold of his ship. When I arrived a dead sailor was being wheeled into x-ray. I asked Dr. Kennedy, 'What do I have to do?' His reply was, 'x-ray him from head to toe. This was for the ship's insurance company. It was a very interesting and rewarding hospital in which to work. We often used our Portugese, Spanish and French dictionaries to help sailors who were far away from their homes. However, in 1950 due to Government changes, the hospital was closed."

Pepperell: Higgins who went to work with the Americans after the war gives some insight into the workings of the military hospital: "Well...Pepperell base was in full swing down there with the Americans and...so I was asked...if I would be interested in working as a civilian nurse on the base and... I took the position and I was there for six years. There were ten air force nurses and only two civilians. According to the agreement with the Government, they had to employ some civilian nurses. They wanted somebody right away because one of the two civilian nurses had gone on vacation and put in her resignation...so they were one short in that way. And it was mostly in a supervisory position because they had the military and the corps men who were like...the student nurses, who were working there. It was in full swing when I went down there. There must have been 5,000 dependants....and that area was called the dependant's area so you did duty there...but you floated then. When the army had clinics, the military personnel did that. But the dependant clinics for tuberculosis and that...we covered...the nurses, even the army nurses, always covered the clinics. We had inspection once a week and they came around...the army did all that...cleaning up for the wards and the area and everything. They came around with white gloves and went along with the white gloves along the tops of the doors and everywhere they could spot. And at that time too, smoking wasn't prohibited like it is today. It wasn't as much of a taboo. And you could go in the utility room and have a smoke. The pay might have been a little bit more but I believe like any jobs that the Newfoundlanders had with the Americans, there was a hold down; they weren't allowed to pay them what they were paying the Americans. The leave was about the same with the Americans and with the military. And I found that we had the responsibility to do a lot of things, like put up IVs and...gave IV medications, it was just another thing to do, where it wasn't permitted if I were working at the General. [You were] a lot more independent there."

Army Reserve: Dewling worked with the Canadian Army, "I did different kinds of nursing; I was in the Army Reserve for a while. I got into that without wanting to go into it. It was at the beginning of the Korean conflict and the medical commanding officer came to see me and told me that he would like me to come up. I told him that I did not want to join the Army, but he asked me to go up and train some nurses for him because none of them up there had any experience with labs. So I went up there to do that and a couple of nights later someone threw a piece of paper at me and I was in the Army and I did not train too many nurses, I did it all myself. It was supposed to be at night. But somehow, the Army made arrangements with the General Hospital because Dr. Roberts came to see me and told me that I had to cooperate with the Army and they will be calling me from time to time and that I had permission to leave when that would happen. I was teaching nursing at the General. So I used to get a call from the switchboard saying that Buckmaster's just called and that there was a car on the way for me. I had my own car, my own driver, and my own list. There were a lot of nurses that went in the Reserve but I don't know any that had all of this. [My husband Art] was a Lieutenant in the British Army and he thought it was absolutely a riot that I had my own driver. It was some years after that that Art and I were at a dance at the Legion and this man kept staring at me. [The man] said that he had not seen me in a long time but he was sure I was the person he thought I was. He asked me if I was Lieutenant Skinner and he said he was my driver for three years."

The *Lady Anderson*: Because of the non existent road system in rural Newfoundland, the sea was the primary route by which health care was brought to the majority of Newfoundlanders. The *Lady Anderson* and the *Christmas Seal* visited communities around Newfoundland on a regular basis. When the ship would arrive the residents of the community went down to the wharf to attend clinics held by the doctor or nurse. The *Lady Anderson* travelled along the south coast of Newfoundland and was equipped to deal with surgical procedures and the administration of anaesthetics. Moakler worked on the *Lady Anderson* where as the only health care provider she diagnosed problems and treated the patients with whatever was available: "And when I went with the Department of Health first, Myrtle Cummings was there and she offered me three positions, two at cottage hospitals and one out on the *Lady Anderson*, so I took the *Lady Anderson*. It was coastal. It was an American yacht of the Newfoundland Government. And they used it out on the coast to get to each of the communities. There was a doctor in Grand Bank and a doctor in Harbour Breton. Other than that, there was no doctor. So we were given all kinds of medications…like a mixture, 'mixed stomatic,' we used to call it for the stomach, or cleanse the chest and if we found that somebody had rales in their chest, you just give him this chest medicine. That was a great job...it was just great. Now how we got our calls was, we would stop say in Harbour Breton, and get a message, a wireless message, saying somebody was very sick in Belleoram so we'd go up to Belleoram. And then when we'd get to Belleoram, there might be another message saying we had to go to Rencontre, and then when you got there...the messages would follow us along the coast. And we'd probably pull in and there'd be eight or ten people waiting on the wharf for us...and the babies, and pulling their teeth and different things. You did very little vaccinations. In those days you were really a medical person. And you'd probably get in somewhere and the people would be further along the road so you'd have to go on horse and sleigh or dog sleigh. I remember one time...it's so vivid in my mind...where we had to go on dog sleigh and it was so treacherous; we were on ice, we were off ice, and I was so glad when I got back on that ship. I must tell you something funny about the captain. Dr. Kent would say to me when we'd go into Harbour Breton, 'The captain had a few drinks today.' But I could never understand how he knew the captain had a few drinks. So when I was leaving the coast, I said to Dr. Kent, 'How did you know when the captain was having a drink?' He said, 'When you'd be coming into Harbour Breton, he would pull one whistle when we were coming in, two whistles if we needed the ambulance, but when he had a few drinks, he used to pull the whistle ham on the ham bone!' He always knew when he had a few drinks. There was a hospital in Harbour Breton and one in Grand Bank. There was a small clinic on the side of the boat and we would look after them there. Yes, I know, no control, when you think about it. It was amazing how many skills you acquired out of necessity. It wasn't unusual; it was expected of you. I felt I was helping somebody and that's what I went in training for."

Gander Airport: Another employer of nurses during that era was the Federal Government at Gander Airport. Gander was the point of entry to North America for transatlantic flights as all flights stopped there for refueling. Anyone wishing to immigrate to Canada or the United States had to have their health documents checked at Gander. Griffen worked at Gander, "I decided to go to National Health and Welfare because you didn't lift or anything. You had regular shifts. I applied and I got the job but I had met Dr. Weisgerber. He was a German and he used to check all their vaccination certificates and, if they weren't vaccinated, they had to be vaccinated then if they wanted to come into the airport. You had to give them vaccinations because we were in cahoots with the States so, they couldn't get into the States because Smallpox was rampant. It might take ten hours, I suppose, or more to come across the Atlantic. And we were really busy. I mean, we'd have 40 flights in the night, it'd be nothing. But probably it's only the same numbers [of passengers] as it is now 'cause the planes were small. Because, at that time, there were a lot of flights coming in with displaced persons...from the war. And nobody ever knew because they were hoarded in the planes like cattle. And at that time, they had bunks in the aircraft. Even the people travelling would pay for a sleeper. If you wake them up and tell them that they weren't vaccinated, they wouldn't get off. They had no intention of getting off after paying a fortune for a berth to come across."

The duties of a nurse in this position included much more than checking for immunizations. Griffen, "And, of course, then if there was babies aboard, we had to make formulas and everything for them. And if any of them ended up in hospital, we looked after them, the National Health, because at one time, they lost a lot of newborns in the hospital; they figured it was somebody who came off the flight with some kind of a germ. They didn't want them to get it again so they would sort of isolate...and we would have to handle it. And if you treated anybody from the States, you'd have to make them sign. One of the girls...somebody had a convulsion and she offered them a doctor. You offer everybody a doctor (laughter) because of the States and he, the person, didn't want a doctor. They said no, they were used to having epileptic seizures and they were fine and months after that, they tried to sue the airlines. And she was asked to go down to [the U.S.] but Dr. Hurdle, because we were under Halifax, said 'No, she didn't have to go.' That's why they couldn't make her go down there to testify."

Nursing for National Health and Welfare afforded many benefits to the nurses. Griffen, "Oh, they hired an awful lot of nurses. It would be about six of us at a time there because there was two on nights there. But in those days, we all lived in the hotel; we didn't stay at the hospital. The nurses at the hospitals stayed at the hospital but we stayed in the hotel. They had a beautiful restaurant, the hotel did. The queerest thing it was, you could come home from work in the morning and, the maids would never touch your room, if you put a sign on, 'you had worked midnights' or 'don't disturb,' they wouldn't touch your room 'til you got up. And you could bring anybody in with you but they had to be out by midnight. Like when I was going out with Des, if he stayed two minutes after midnight, they called the ones in charge of C.Q. and she'd be checking to make sure that everybody was out. And, not only that, when we worked with National Health and Welfare, we made more money than most nurses in Newfoundland. We got the nurse's rate on the mainland. And we were called category three. Now, after a couple of months, you went to category three which was the highest paid. Oh it was fantastic! Our meals were included. And the meals we ate in the terminal, we sent in…you know, we kept receipts and we got paid for them. And our uniforms were free. I mean, first we wore naval uniforms. And then after that, they changed, they had a black and white one and then finally we had red. By the time I left, we had red uniforms but we wore white coats over…like we took off the jacket, but boarding the aircraft, you had to wear your red."

Working in Gander meant there was a lot of cooperation between the members of the medical team and the flight crew. Griffen, "Another night, they had a flight and they had this man in the back seat of the plane and he was just like this, you know (demonstrating to interviewer). The captain said, 'Don't say anything about that, you know, because he's dead. But we're going to leave him here on the seat, but don't tell anybody, because when we get airborne and get near New York, we'll say we have a passenger who died.' Yeah, so that's what they did. They took off and when they got near New York, or wherever they were landing, they called and said they had a passenger…because, see if they died here, they'd have to take him and put him in a steel casket and all that kind of stuff…and the whole plane would be held for ages!"

In fact some of the situations that Griffen found herself in were dangerous. Griffen, "Now this night, they had a flight that came from Saudi Arabia and they hadn't seen a woman for months. Anyhow, first of all, some of them weren't vaccinated and we had to vaccinate them. And they were so rowdy and everything that the mountie came up to stay with us while we were vaccinating them. So we heard this ruckus outside and the stewardess runs in, and she says 'Oh, come out, come out, there's somebody bleeding!' And I said, 'Call your captain. Don't go telling me.' And she said, 'No, come on, you got to go.' So anyhow, I had to call the doctor into the hospital. So he came up, and I'll never forget it. So anyhow, he just gave him an injection and he assured him that he'd sleep, but the flight got delayed. So buddy started waking up. So they came in and said, 'He's awake.' And the captain said, 'Look, he's awake, what are we going to do?' So I called the doctor again. He said, 'Joan, I'm not coming up.

Go out and give him an injection and make sure you give him enough that either it kills him or he sleeps.' So I went out, and the mountie was a real small man, and he said, 'I'll go aboard the aircraft with you.' So when I went out, he [the passenger] went to grab me, and the mountie struck him right here somewhere on his neck (demonstrating) and laid him out a cold junk. Yes, the mountie hit him right here when he went to grab me and he said, 'He won't wake up, Joan, 'til he gets to New York, for sure.' But I still gave him the injection to make sure, so I don't know; we didn't hear that he died (laughter)."

In the 1950s, Gander was known as the 'Crossroads of the World,' and consequently had its share of famous visitors, all of whom had to be checked by the nurse. However, Griffen was not deterred by their fame. Griffen relates a few stories about her brushes with fame, 'Well, sure when Guggarin, who was the first man in space...I wasn't working but Chris Dunne, she graduated from the Grace...she was working and she was a character. Anyhow, they landed in Gander, it was on a Saturday or Sunday...she couldn't get hold of Halifax, and they landed in Gander. He wasn't vaccinated. Now he had come back from space so she wasn't allowed to let him off. So he was very short, apparently, so she came down off the flight and she said, 'That's a sin. That poor little fella all dressed up in his new uniform and he can't get off.' Well the news heard about him, because everybody knew he was landing here. There were news people everywhere. They wanted her to go on whatever program it was they used to interview people, like on CBC in those days. But she wouldn't go. And the only one I ever had trouble with was Hugh Hefner with his bunny plane. He didn't think anybody should board that because he had a gorgeous bed in it and everything like that. He was some disgusted 'til he found out he couldn't land and he wouldn't be allowed to do anything in Gander unless the nurses cleared him, so he had to let us aboard. That's the only fella I had trouble with. And one night...the movie actors used to come in on a flight and I was clearing the flight this night and, Frankie Sinatra was on it. So I asked him for his vaccination certificate and he said, 'You show me yours.' And I said, 'We're vaccinated.' And I had a long talk to him and Sammy Davis Jr. was with him, and I never went to movies very much, so I didn't know who I was talking to anyhow (laughter). So one of the men said, 'You had some talk to Frankie, Joan.' And I said, 'Who? Is Frankie Broderick working?' They said, 'Who did you think you were just talking to? Frank Sinatra, my dear, that's who!' It pays to be ignorant, doesn't it? And another time the flight was cancelled here and

Sean, my oldest boy, said, 'Oh mom, there's…. oh, the English fella now I can't remember his name…get his autograph.' I said, 'Sean, I'm not starting that racket getting autographs; there's no way am I going to do it.' And so anyhow Sutherland kept coming back and forth into the office, and finally I said, 'Do you want a cup of coffee?' He said, 'Sure.' I said, 'I don't know what you're doing here coming back and forth in here.' He said, 'But you've got personality; I've never met anybody as friendly as you are.' So in the meantime, Sean called. He said, 'Mom, change your mind. That whole plane is filled with movie stars.' I said, 'I'll see what I can do for you.' So I came out and I said to buddy, 'Do you know Donald Sutherland on the flight? And he said, 'Yes.' And I said, 'My son…you know, if I were that nice to give you a cup of coffee…my son would like an autograph.' 'That's no problem,' he said 'who do you think I am?' I said, 'I haven't got two clues.' He said, 'That's who I am, Donald Sutherland.' And he gave….the autograph. So Pearl Romley was from the mainland, and she loved movies. So Customs said, 'You missed it today, my dear, 'cause Joan is out giving coffee.' So she called and she said, 'Joan, are you sure the cup and saucer matched?' I said, 'My dear, he had coffee Newfie style; I don't care what matched. I couldn't tell you'."

As today, opportunities in the nursing profession were so broad that nurses could find their niche in jobs that challenged their interests and abilities. Their work also provided circumstances where they flourished and used their skills to respond to the needs of the agency and their patients.

PART 3 :

The Outside World & Other Influences

The focus of the interviews was the nursing careers of these nurses however in reviewing the data it quickly became evident that the participants, their recollections and stories had to be viewed within the context of the world in which they lived and worked. These women lived through world wars and other historical events which impacted directly on their environment and their practice. Their stories revealed the socioeconomic conditions of the time, the resulting social issues and health problems and the implications for health care delivery. They entered nursing when communicable diseases were rampant, antibiotics were non-existent, poverty commonplace and society's expectations of women were vastly different from today. The participants' recollections provide insight into their world of nursing, the relationship between nurses and doctors as well as the many challenges they faced both as women and as nurses. This section looks at the impact of war, of Confederation, and of disease both on the population and on the nurses. It also explores a society where women were required to leave the workplace if they married, where accessability to health care was not guaranteed and where nurses played a significantly different role in health care delivery from that of today.

CHAPTER 9:
Environmental Influences

"I remember when they torpedoed...off Cape Spear or out there...and they came in...[it was] terrible and when I think of war now...it's a horrible thing." Barrett (41)

"It [Confederation] changed the whole thing...they got better housing...when I think of going up to some of those houses...literally mud on the floor...the whole thing changed. [People's living conditions] improved tremendously." Penney (45)

World War II: Although Newfoundland was far from the front in World War II, the province did not escape its impact. Fourteen of the participants graduated from nursing between 1939 and 1945 so it was not surprising that the war was a significant piece of their nursing career. Their stories reflected what life was like in St. John's during that period as well as the horrors of war. These women also revealed how the war impacted them and their work world particularly when sharing their memories of the victims.

Nurses were responsible for the preparations for the blackout which existed throughout the war in addition to their regular nursing duties. Tobin outlined her duties as a student nurse, "Of course, then the war was on and there were the blackouts that we would have to prepare for. There was a board that we would fit into the window at around 4:00 p.m. each evening and that would stay there until daylight the next day." Barrett, "We had great big shutters, the size of the window. And made out of plywood. And every single afternoon when it began to get dark, every shutter had to go up. We had to put up...I had to put up my shutter in my bedroom. And that was up all night." Penney "I was at the Fever then and we had to close the wooden windows. We had the wooden shutters... and you couldn't let any light get out...that was all part of the war years. You had to be very careful when you were out yourself, of course, in the blackout (laughing). The Sisters would always say to us, the last words practically going out, 'Just watch where you're going.' I mean the soldiers and sailors (laughing)." Bruce, "We brought in our ration books when we came in and they were passed in [to the hospital]. Ration books went around during the war. That allowed them to get you your food supply?" Moakler, "Because we trained during the war, they [the clocks] had two hours on instead of that one hour so it was light at 10:00 o'clock. I mean, we had to be in bed at 10:00 o'clock and we'd look out through the window and we could hear the kids down playing hopscotch...we had to be in bed because...the house mother would make rounds." Ashbourne, "In '43, they started to...give the students $5.95 a month. The student's first cheque was referred to as a war bonus."

Within the health care system, the impact of war was evident particularly in the delivery of services and availability of resources. Story, "After I finished grade 11, I worked as a nursing assistant and that was in 1942 and 1943. There was still war on the go then. But they took the ladies' side of Memorial University and turned it into a hospital for the Merchant seamen and I was there for nine months." Strong, "I was in charge [at the Waterford] from 1942 to 1949. Dr Charlie Roberts went to the Army but when the war was over he came back as Superintendent." Penney gives some idea as to the impact of the doctor's absence on patient care, "I'd love to study it, psychiatry, but at that time when I was there [at the Waterford]...they didn't have a doctor there...the doctor had gone off to war really. You didn't have too much direction...but then they would call in a doctor if they had a need, or they felt there was a need. There wasn't really a lot of going on there in the way of treatment."

The military personnel stationed in St. John's were treated by their own doctors and did not usually avail of health care services in the St. John's hospitals. Avery, "There was a military hospital on the base. It was very seldom if we did [have soldiers as patients], because they had their own hospital." Mifflin, "I remember this chap came in one day. Apparently someone had thrown an axe at him and he had a cut right across his forehead. Now, we were not supposed to have anything to do with the soldiers, if they came in you had to send them back to the barracks. We would call the barracks and someone would come and pick them up. Anyway this chap came in with the cut on his forehead. I put a dressing on it for him and called his barracks. They had their own doctors. Unless they were dying we would have to send them back."

Of course, there also were the social benefits of having a large contingent of soldiers housed in the city. Moakler, "And the thing about training was we loved to dance, we loved to sing, and downstairs in the nursing home, at that time, was a big hall where we had our dances and...we'd take up the phone and just phone down to the base and say we needed X number of men and we'd have all these soldiers that would come up from the base. It was just great! Innocent fun! And, if they phoned and they'd say, 'We need two girls or three girls to go out tonight.' The house mother would say, 'Well you better come up 'til I have a look at you first.' And she would decide who was going out with these men...they didn't phone you...it was the house mother." Penney, "Of course...thousands of them [soldiers] were here then. There was partying but we didn't get to do much of that...I was there VJ Day. I remember...it was quite, quite the thing." Avery, "We had a lot of soldiers come around the hospital because they were dating nurses and a lot of them married. We had one wander into the residence one night and came up on the floor. He crawled into a bed in the same room with a nurse...[who] didn't have much on because she was sleeping. The soldier was drinking and ended up just going to sleep. She could not get up to go and call anyone because she didn't have enough clothes on; she was afraid. One of the nurses came by and helped her. They ended up getting the soldier up and led him out the door. We were very glad about that."

The most significant memories of the war for these women were the war victims in their care. Barrett, "I remember when they torpedoed...off Cape Spear or out there. And they came...I was on Carson Ward on night duty, and one had gas gangrene. [The ship was torpedoed and it was one of the Canadian men]. Several men came in that night. And the doctors were all back and everything. And you could hear the gas...and you could hear the gas escaping [out of his limbs]. His hands in particular. He died...terrible and when I think of war now it's a horrible thing." Sister Fabian, "During the war, we had a lot of emergencies. I remember one night we admitted 11 or 12 who had been out on the high seas for days and some of them ended up losing their limbs. That night we had to make an office into a room, so we could put extra people in there. [Only a couple of] doctors were there to take care of them...they were seamen and were probably shipwrecked." Ashbourne, "In '42 we had tragedies because it was just after we graduated when the Germans torpedoed just off Bell Island. We were called back in. It was rushed. Rush! Rush! Rush! They all had to be fixed...like a lot of burns...and a lot of people had succumbed to the fire." Tobin, "We were in charge of a unit. There were 29 beds and I think Carson was the worst one. This was during the war so, not only did you have your 29 beds but you could have three or four narrow cots that were put in between the beds. These were survivors of torpedoes, burns or whatever. Carson was Urology so they would be placed in between all of these patients." Penney, "We got the odd sailors in…we never knew from where but I guess from boats outside."

Not all the victims of the war resulted from action. Avery recalls a young soldier far away from home: "Another soldier came into the nursery one night and tried to leave with a baby. There were two of us on that night, Mrs. Benson and myself. Mrs. Benson is the night supervisor. I ran for her and Newton held him back and talked to him. When Mrs. Benson came over, he told her that his wife in the States had a baby that day and he was only up to look at the babies. He said he needed a baby for the night. So, she told him that he could not have a baby but she talked to him about his baby in the States and he went on his way."

Probably the most horrifying experience of the war for these women was the fire at the Knights of Columbus in December, 1942. Four of the participants discussed the fire, three of whom were first year students (in nursing only four to six months) and a new graduate. Their vivid recollections tell of the horror of that night, particularly from the perspective of the health care workers. Avery, "The K of C fire was…the first night that I was on the door. I was getting pretty well past being a probationer at that time. It was around 10:00 o'clock when the housemother ran down and said that the barn dance just went off the air. The two of us ran out into the street and we could see the flames shooting into the air from the building that was way down LeMarchant Road and then on Harvey Road. There was a bend in the road but we could still see the flames. We went back and went upstairs, we locked the door and stood on chairs looking out over the corner of the hospital and we could see the flames. We were only there about five minutes and we could hear the ambulances coming. In no time the hospitals were filled. They had patients on the floor and everywhere. The people who were on that night said that people just crawled out of their skin where they were so burnt. People died on the floor and everything. When we left to go over to the hospital in the morning there was a stench of burnt hair and flesh in the residence and through the tunnel. Over at the hospital it was a very gray morning. Wherever there was space to put a bed or a cot there was somebody in it. After a few days they died or they were put somewhere where they could be treated, other than in a corridor. We had some of them for months, treating them and looking after them until they were well enough to leave. Some of them were really sick with really big burns. We did burn dressings for weeks on end. On the day of the fire, in the afternoon when we got off for a couple of hours, myself and one of the other nurses, walked down and the fire was still smoldering. Everything was leveled to the ground. I don't know if they got all of the bodies or not. For weeks people were being buried and things were being cleaned up. It went on and on; it was a real tragedy." Penney, "The K of C. That night! Oh my! You know, they brought them…to St. Clare's. It was the nearest hospital… and we were just students just in; that was in, I believe…'42. And we were all rushed out of bed to go over and do our bit. It was terrible. All those people were so badly burned, you know. Most…a lot of them died…and a lot of them were dead that were brought in. But I remember they didn't take…they took some of them but you know it was the space. They shared out some, I think, with the General but…St. Clare's was so close to it." Moakler, "I was in training when the K of C fire started and walking through the corridors the morning after the K of C fire, the stench of burned bodies…I think I can still smell it. [I was] a student nurse, just in training. Most of the patients were dispersed to the bigger wards. I remember one patient, badly burned in the face. I wouldn't know him now if he came in the door because I never saw him with his bandages off, but his name was Mark Anthony, and that stands in my mind. I have no idea of where he is or what he did but I spent a lot of time with that young fella. And, as I said, I often wonder where he is or what he did afterwards." Sister Fabian, "Yes I remember that [the K of C fire], it was a terrible night. We had people brought to us that we had no beds for. We treated them with first aid and they were transferred to the General; we did not have anybody long term from that fire. We had a little student nurse on duty that night and her brother was killed in that fire. She worked all night and did not know what had happened to him until the next morning. She knew that he was there but she did not know his status."

The victim impact of the war extended well beyond its end. Griffen who worked with National Health and Welfare (at Gander Airport), "Nobody could board the aircraft 'til the nurses boarded and cleared it. There was a lot of flights coming in with displaced persons (DPs)…from the war.…if they didn't get in to the States by 5:00 o'clock… Friday, there would be no Red Cross or anything on duty so they'd have to spend time in Gander in the hotels. And nobody ever knew because they were like hoarded in the planes like cattle and...I remember one baby died in a room. Of course, they didn't want to let anybody know that anybody was sick. Because they wouldn't get into the States, they were so scared; they were really pitiful. I called him [the doctor] but we didn't know who owned the baby because nobody would admit to it, you know...they were afraid they wouldn't get into the States. They used to bring their x-rays and...then he [the doctor] did a physical on them before they could go on. Displaced persons who were coming as immigrants...probably be 50 or something on the plane. They'd come about once a week. They were pitiful people because they were so scared...they were going to the States ninety percent of them, and we only had to check their vaccinations. It was only the ones going to Canada, the immigrants going to Canada, that we would have to...do a good physical on them."

Woodland related several stories which tell of the local aftermath of the war. She and one other girl made up the 1945 class entering nursing at the Grace: "There was just the two of us [in the class]...it was post-war...and they couldn't get anybody to come in training....getting married, most of them...and material was hard to get. So I ended up having secondhand uniforms. I had somebody else's name on all my uniforms. (laughter). And we could only wear...one blue dress a week, and four aprons and bibs. So what you did, you wore the apron on one side for one day and put it on the other side for the next day (laughter)! It was nothing for us to have 10 and 15 babies a night. You know, men came here from overseas and everybody had a baby. We used to have them in the corridors on stretchers...at night. What we used to do in the Case Room, the ones that were delivered, we didn't have a bed for them downstairs and we'd put them in what we used to call the small OR where they'd do the tonsillectomies and everything. And in the morning at 7:00 o'clock, you'd have to drag all these stretchers out in the corridor again (laughter) so they could do their OR work again. And it was terrible really...when you stop to think."

Career Interruptions: An individual's career in nursing might be interrupted for one of two reasons: illness (personal or family) or marriage. They worked in an environment rampant with communicable diseases and where effective treatments such as antibiotics were nonexistent. They lived in an era when women did not usually work outside the home once they married. It was also commonplace that a daughter would interrupt (or give up) her career to care for a family member who was ill. Through their stories we get a real sense of the different world of nursing in which they worked and the sacrifices they were prepared and sometimes expected to make.

Tuberculosis (Tb): Tuberculosis was rampant in Newfoundland during the time that these women practiced nursing. As a result they were a vulnerable population and it is not surprising that many of them succumbed to the disease. Barron, "I was doing a rotation in the operating room and because it was Good Friday there was no surgery and they decided to do chest x-rays on student nurses. I had a chest x-ray and on the following Tuesday...the call came...Sister Catherine wants you in her office and I thought *Oh, my God*. I never got into any trouble. I knew I hadn't broken any of the rules. The only thing I could think of was that someone was dead belong to me or I had Tb. Sure it was like the bottom came away, one of the worse things, just like telling you had terminal cancer...the same reaction. They tell you there was a chance, I know there's always a chance but things were desperate then...I just couldn't handle it. I think I stayed two or three days. I don't know how I told them at home, I don't know because my brother had died. Anyway I went home because if I went to the San I had to wait for a bed and it was silly to wait for a bed so I went home to Ferryland instead and it was six weeks before I started. I went out for graduation...they wanted me to graduate with the class. I didn't want to...I always wanted to finish before and to me I wasn't finished...I went there because I was told to. I couldn't go to my dance...I didn't get to that and you know I always miss that. By this time most of the girls had their RNs...that was pretty upsetting. And then that day while I was there I talked to Dr. Brownrigg and I said, 'Can you get me into the San?' So I think they got a bed around the 26th of January. Well it took artificial pneumothorax. My lung was 75% collapsed for two years and I went back. There was a lot of anxiety, [I had no guarantee] whether I'd get back...PAS and INAH came out...now I wasn't on any of that at that point but before I left there I had a course of Streptomycin...I had strep every day...and I just had six weeks of that and PAS and INAH. They let me go home on bathroom privileges because they used to keep you in and because I was a nurse, that made a difference too. They considered you more safe...instead of keeping me in I was allowed to go home on half exercises for a while and then get up in the chair and do full exercises. So I had to follow what I was supposed to do at home. [My lung] was collapsed when I finished training."

Oakley, "I graduated in 1931 and the last six months I was in the Operating Room and I had a bad hip then. They took an x-ray and I ended up going to bed for a year. They said I had a Tb hip. I was not sick or anything but they would not let me go home. They put me into one of the Salvation Army homes here because I was an officer at the time. I think I shed buckets of tears when I went in there; I wanted to be [a] nurse. To think that I had just graduated and now I was crippled. I graduated and then went on holidays, which ended up to be a year because we had no Orthopedic doctor and [the doctor] used to come from Halifax. I was in that home for eight months and they were very good to me. I had a 13 pound weight on my leg that they took off in May. I was in the bed for the full eight months. After they took the weight off, they were going to put a cast on but where it was so much better, they let me go home on crutches. Anyway, I went back to Grand Bank and in August, [the doctor] came down from Halifax and sent a message to me to come for an examination and an x-ray...I could walk with a stick then. Dr. Anchor asked Dr. Roberts if the x-rays belong to that girl. So, they concluded that there was nothing wrong with me then."

Several other participants reported having classmates who had contracted tuberculosis during training and could not finish their program. Not just students were vulnerable but all nurses, whether they worked in that environment or not. Barrett, "E. Belle Rogers [Director of Nursing], took sick with Tb...and she received nursing care in the residence until she went to a sanatorium on the mainland, and Dr. Brownrigg went with her." French reported that when she first went to work at the Sanatorium in 1944, several of the nursing staff contracted Tb, but "Dr. Brownrigg was very annoyed by that." Apparently he took steps to try and reduce the nurses' risk. Griffen, "One of the girls from my class ended up in the San...she got Tb. So Doctor Brownrigg had said no wonder we had Tb because we're in germs all day and we were never allowed to get out anymore. So they decided then you had...to take a...half hour when you came off but you had to get out of your uniform...and you had to go outdoors...and (laughter) then you had to get back in your uniform and get back to work and all in a half hour. So we used to hide away as best as we could so we wouldn't have to go outdoors. So it didn't help."

Other Communicable Diseases: Tuberculosis wasn't the only threat to the students' well being and some spent time at the Fever Hospital, not just as students but as patients. Any time missed from the nursing program had to be paid back before the students could graduate. Griffen, "I spent time down there [at the Fever] because that's where I had Diphtheria...and that's how I got Endocarditis from the Diphtheria. [It was tough] especially when I had my RN and was still putting in sick time." Moakler, "I also spent time at the Fever when I was in training...I was just due to go on holidays that morning and woke up so I took it. [That delayed my training] and, of course, you had to make it up. You had to make up any time that you had off sick." Avery, "I was down there [at the Fever] with the Mumps. They had them [Mumps] down at the Grace and they cleaned up the whole crowd and carbolized everything. They had the rooms that the student nurses were in painted and everything. I would go over and give candy to all of the students with Mumps. They were patients in an isolated room. I thought I was beyond getting Mumps...I ended up with the Mumps. They sent me to the Fever."

The occurrence of communicable diseases, particularly Tb and Polio was not an isolated event and often occurred in epidemic proportions. As a public health nurse, Avery gives some idea as to the measures taken to prevent the spread of and eradicate communicable diseases in the province. "We did a lot of Tb tests and vaccinations for Tb. During the Polio years, we would have Polio clinics and they would be lined up through the door; people would become very frustrated because they could not get in any faster. We could not get them in any faster because it would be too warm and too many people in the room. After the tests and vaccinations, we would have to boil all of the needles because they did not come packaged and sterilized back then. The problem with that was, we were not given enough to do us. So, I would have to ask one of the ladies that was there if she would wash and boil the needles for me. Of course I would show her how to do it. I would have to take them from the pot and put them into a sterile towel and use them over again...at the Polio clinic. The whole community would be done. Nobody wanted it but it had to be done. People would even come to my house because they worked in the day and you couldn't feel guilty you had to do it. Sometimes they would be there in your house before you knew what you were doing. The Polio time was a real scare. We vaccinated at all of the schools for Polio, Diptheria, and Whooping Cough."

Family Illness: Family illness was also sufficient reason for a student or graduate to interrupt her career and return home to care for a family member. House, "I wanted to give it up [working in Corner Brook] and I phoned Mom and found out that she had been ordered to rest...I think she was upset that I left. But my father died the year before and I left home and...she said 'If you want to come...come on...I'm not very well.' So that decided me right then." French, "I graduated just as the war started. I went home because my mother was sick and never went back to work until 1944. [The matron] would call to know when I was coming back to work. When I returned I went to the Sanatorium on Topsail Road." Dalley, "Mom got sick; I had to come home. And I was home...I had to take care of her all that time [over six months]." Williams, "I was only in there seven months, just after getting my cap, when my mother got sick. And I had to go home. So while I was home, she died. So Major Fagner...the Superintendent there [at the Grace], she phoned me...or wired, and told me to be back on duty then as soon as possible. That's what my mother died with [Tb]. Not the lungs...[the doctor] told me she had two Tb kidneys. I was only seven months in training – when I came home to look after her, she said, 'Ethel, I'm some proud you went in for nursing. You can do some little things now to help me out.' I didn't know very much at seven months...but still, I knew how to make her bed and I knew how to wash her, bath her, and she didn't mind me doing a thing for her." Ashbourne, "I went back [to Twillingate]...well, my mother had surgery and I went back then to be with her."

Marriage: The married nurse working in a hospital was an unknown phenomena in the 1930s and 40s although there were some changes in the 1950s. If a nurse got married, she was required to quit her job in the hospital, although the participants' stories suggest there was plenty of work for married and pregnant women doing private duty. Whiteway, "I left in 1943...I got married...and you had to leave. [You weren't allowed to work]." Strong, "In 1949 I got married; I could not work after I was married back then." Merrigan, "[I worked] one year. Then I got married. [I worked after I got married] but only 3 months. I got pregnant right away. I worked for a while until they started marking me. I stopped work because I was pregnant...most women did that then. They wouldn't be caught working." Ashbourne, "I went back in October and got married...we had to [quit]...you weren't allowed to work." Bruce, "I don't know if there was ever a rule [about getting married] but it just was not done. That is not one hundred percent either because when my last child was born [1959] I worked out of the nursing office until I was well along in pregnancy. But it was unusual...I don't remember any rule. It just was not done." Nurse, "I'm probably the first married nurse down at that level, I think. And I went down...went in after my honeymoon of a weekend and saw Mary Feehan to say that I was married and I was hoping I wasn't going to be fired on the spot. And I worked up right to my pregnancy. Of course, nobody knew I was pregnant (laughter)." Barron, "Oh God, no! you weren't allowed to work after you got married (laughing). Oh my dear, if you were pregnant you might as well go kill yourself. But I mean, you know, that was out of the question. A nurse...a married nurse didn't even ask to work, it was just taken for granted you didn't. So I don't even know if you asked, if they'd say yes." Woodland, "I got married and moved to Grand Falls. I didn't work... they didn't employ married women, the A and D Company, at that time. That was a policy. The A and D Company owned and ran the hospital. So they didn't employ married women even in the mill, the office staff or anything. Once you got married, that was it – you were out (laughter). But I could go in and relieve if somebody got sick, or had a baby or something like that, you know?" By the mid 1950s there was a change in attitude. King, "I got married in 1955. I was on a six month leave of absence without pay and then I came back to work. I returned to the same position. [To have my children] I did the same thing. I took a leave of absence. I never resigned [from nursing]." As more married nurses entered the work force, it became an advantage in some cases. Penney worked with public health in St. John's; "I had gotten married ...and you didn't have to go out of town if you were married and the girls that were single didn't appreciate it."

Pre and Post Confederation: One of the beliefs underlying this project was that nursing would be different pre and post Confederation. While only a few of the participants actually referred to Confederation, many of them did refer to living conditions in the province prior to Confederation and for some years following. Their stories provide valuable insight into the socioeconomic circumstances of the people (in some cases well into the mid 1960s) and the significance for nursing practice. The stories tell of the poverty that existed throughout the province, the health problems arising from that poverty, the difficulty people had in accessing health care as well as the difficulties nurses encountered in their attempts to care for their patients. Alternatly, they tell of the positive changes that occurred as a result of Confederation both for the people and for nurses.

Socioeconomic Conditions: The average Newfoundlander would find it difficult today to understand that prior to Confederation there was a segment of the population who lived in what could be best described as third world conditions. Poverty was a province wide issue. Nurses working in the community were the ones who dealt primarily with this group as most could not afford to pay for health care and subsequently relied on the public health nurse to come to them or they went to the public health clinics. Taylor who worked on the coast: "They weren't really too well off. People just didn't have very much really. [There wasn't any fruit]. I mean you might get...oranges and apples on the coastal boat. They didn't give you very much and...[it] was all canned goods." For most of the nurses working in the community it was the impact on the children that they recalled most vividly. Moakler, "I did the schools...I can't believe it now, but there were so many dirty heads. Children were going to school with their heads shaved with bandanas tied around them, because of lice...and it seemed to me like that's all we did in schools then...was just check heads...very poor hygiene! Of course, the homes didn't have running water. A lot of them didn't have...indoor toilets or anything. It's interesting [but] you have to blame a lot of it on us because we knew what we were doing. I remember years ago, we moved people from...I forget the name of that place there now...we moved them there...and we didn't tell them about the bathtub, or the toilet, or the sink, and when we went back, they had coal in the bathtub because they didn't know what the bathtub was for! So we have to blame ourselves for that. [There was no such thing as health teaching in those days]." Hutchings who worked on the Northern Peninsula encountered the same hygiene problems in the school and the homes as her counterparts in St. John's: "You must remember in most of these homes until well into the 60s they didn't have any running water. So I mean it was difficult to keep the children clean." Measures to improve the health of children began at birth. Godden who worked with Child Welfare, "We'd talk to the mother about the baby...if she breastfed or what formula she would have...and if the baby's stomach was healed...when to serve solid food...and advise her about coming to the well baby clinic. [The clinics] were just for children...from birth up to five years. The doctor would advise us to provide the mother with milk ...and cod liver oil and orange juice...provided from the Government...and given out at the clinic. We gave the orange juice as an incentive...concentrated orange juice. Every afternoon was open for immunizations – Whooping Cough, Diptheria and Tetanus – we did it at the clinic and the nurses went around the homes and did it."

Penney, "It [Confederation] changed the whole thing. They got better housing...when I think of going up to some of those houses...literally mud on the floor. The whole thing changed. [People's living conditions] improved tremendously. And...we'd have to do the school in the district or there might be several. And the hygiene was terrible for the children. The Pediculi were something else. Everyone covered [with lice] and impetigo...and all the things that poor hygiene, and poor housing and... three or four of them in the one bed. And if one got it they all got it. And after Confederation...the children had better hygiene and better clothing and whatnot. The housing was so much improved. Because even when they got the housing in the center of town...we moved some of those. I moved them, physically...because some of them were patients and we helped move the patients themselves when the houses were ready. I'm trying to think what they called it then. But they all moved up. That was the big move from the center of the town and from really poor housing and it was the first time that they had the facilities...you know, bathroom facilities and water, because they used to come out to the pump, and get the water out on the street and come to the center of the town in those days. And put their slop pails, as they used to say, out at night, to be picked up. So it took them a little while to adjust because...they didn't respect it first but then they got used to it, and it was marvelous. That was a great, great improvement."

"[We would do a delivery at home after Confederation] if a person wanted to stay home, but as we got more, I guess, more beds or whatever, in the hospitals, I think the doctor would suggest to them...we had our anti-natal clinic and our doctor was there, an obstetrician and...if he saw, or he thought, that there was going to be a difficulty or something, he'd advise them to go to hospital. I'm talking back fifty years...and they just didn't have even the most menial things. You went in...they didn't have anything ready for the baby and you were possibly in two rooms and there were possibly three or four more in the kitchen or the bedroom...in some of the poorer areas. They were even in the center of the city sometimes...I remember putting them in the box down in the kitchen drawer. They had the babies...taking the blanket off the bed and some of them would put it there...but some of them were really good. And you were delivering possibly in the bedroom and with a piece of material pulled across because there may not be a door. I remember that. With possibly bed bugs running up the side of the wall (laughing). And then the children...a couple of children were out on what they used to call, the coal box, in the kitchen. And the father trying to keep some kind of a fire...in the kitchen...to keep it warm. But...they did well. I don't know if it cost in the hospital or if that was the way they wanted to do it...because they had to be home. The father had to go to work or whatever, if he was working, which many times he wasn't…to be home with the children and… that was it. And they breastfed; they all breastfed. And, you know, they never got infections. Of course, some of the old doctors used to tell us, you just leave them in their own. If you don't introduce anything new…it's all right. They'd do well." According to Woodland, in the early 1950s there were still women in the city who delivered their babies at home: "Dr. Roberts used to go out on maternity cases because he'd often come and get one of the Grace grads to go with him. He did do some home deliveries. He would just come in and say 'I need a nurse' and…whoever was off duty would go but you didn't get paid for it! They were welfare cases."

Transportation and communications were major issues in health care delivery both pre and immediately post Confederation. Roche, "Back then, especially in the 60s transportation was terrible…[we would travel however we could]. There was a coastal boat or a helicopter to bring you out or the patient in. We did not use telephones then. We used telegraph." Hutchings, "There's like two parts of nursing. When I was isolated and after the road came. I think the road was a deal made [with Confederation]. In 1956 the road came as far as St. Paul's…we were still isolated until 1962…you couldn't really plan things.. But after the bridge went in to St Paul's and…to Parsons Pond…you could go and…say now I'm going to do…I had a set thing…I did my sterilizations. First I had to put the packs I needed sterile into the oven with a potato…and when the potato was cooked…it was sterile. But I asked the department for a pressure cooker so I was able to do some stuff in the pressure cooker. And then when we got the road and there was someone going back and forth I'd send them up to Bonne Bay and they did the sterilization for me up there." Taylor talked of the isolation working on the coast; "You'd talk to them [other nurses] by radio telephone…and occasionally the nurse…from Flower's Cove came for a few days…that was rare…unusual."

Accessability to Health Care: The biggest barrier to health care delivery in the province was accessability. Many of the respondents told of their practice experiences and the lengths they took to care for their patients. However, even if the nurse, doctor, or health service was on hand not all of the citizens could avail of them. Barron, "I can't say there was any big changes in the period of time [after Confederation] because people still …had to pay for their rooms [in hospital]. They had to pay for everything. If they took an aspirin we had to document it. You had to chart everything that a person had so the day they were going home that list was sent down to nursing office for insurance." Payment for health care was also an issue when Barron provided services in the community: "You had to pay for all your services...I don't know if you could get a doctor without paying for it. People having to go to hospital or go to a doctor, it would cost them money. So they called me and I think it was great because I was home and could go." Merrigan, "If you had an emergency, you had to call the doctor and sometimes the doctor would ask if there would be money in it for him. [They were not paid by Medicare then]. The first thing he did was ask for the money before he would come out...[but] he would come out."

Sister Fabian, "Because it was a private operation; we did not have any public patients besides children. Then, for a while we had a special bursary that some of the parishes supported, for poor mothers who wanted to come to St. Clare's; therefore they were not considered Public Health because they were getting paid. We had that from the 40s until we went into health insurance. Of course, it wasn't necessary then because everybody could get paid. But there were still some poor mothers coming and the doctors in the first year of health insurance were not covered. I believe MCP came out a year later. So the money that was in that burse then went towards paying the doctors to take care of them. Some of the parishes used to give money along with friends of the hospital. After I trained, Dr. Miller was the only pediatrician in St John's and he wasn't in practice, only public health. Every Sunday morning he used to come in and have a look at the children; we had a lot of the poor children at that time and they came from all around. The rest of the patients at that time were private patients who were paying his or her own way; there was no health insurance."

Giovannini, "We did a monthly report and sent it in as well as, order our medications. I must say, the Government back then was very generous; I used to sell Aspirin for 10 cents per dozen. They would have to pay for their own. There was not the Welfare that there is today. [You collected the money and would have to send it in]...they would have to pay for their own and they knew that; if they did not pay, they did not get it. They did not have a lot of money but those days, the hospitals used to have an annual fee of $15.00, which was sort of like MCP. But if you could not pay it but had a big garden, you could pay in kind. You could pay with so many sacks of potatoes or sacks of vegetables or even pay with milk. Of course, I did an occasional midwifery [and] they paid $10.00. I used to charge 25 cents to pull a tooth."

In addition to the social changes that came from Confederation, there were changes for nurses both in their practice and in the educational opportunities. Tobin, "After Confederation there were changes. There were graduates in charge then. It changed then because we went from a 12 hour shift to the 8 hour shift. Then you had a registered nurse between the units and the students did not have the responsibilities then, as they would have had." Roche, "There were no standards. As a student you had a procedure book and that is what you went by. Eventually someone brought out policy manuals for nursing. That was in the 50s. It was started by nurses who went to the mainland universities. It was what the trends were up there and they would bring them home." Joining Confederation pointed out other differences in nursing in Newfoundland and on the 'mainland.' Avery, "I went away [to Toronto] and I was just a general nurse, I didn't have my RN. So I had a choice of writing or wait until the next year for Newfoundland to join Canada. But I didn't know that Newfoundland was going to join Canada, so I wrote the exam and passed." Moakler, "That year we entered into Canada, I was at the University of Toronto…and I know that up there they used to say, 'Oh, you'll soon be Canadians now, you'll be a lot better off.' Now that didn't sit very well with us up there. And then we were amazed when we'd go to class and they'd say, 'If you had a patient who was ready to deliver, what would you do?' Now I mean, my thing was deliver them because we delivered them! But they were horrified with that, because they didn't do that on the mainland…you had to get them to the hospital regardless."

Newfoundland nurses were traveling out of country to universities for further education prior to Confederation. For example, at St Clare's Hospital many of the Sisters did additional education programs in the United States after they completed their nursing program to prepare them for roles in the hospital, such as nurse anesthetist, but also to teach the nursing students. Strong went to Toronto in 1949 to complete a one year post graduate program in psychiatric nursing before returning to work as a staff nurse at the Hospital for Mental and Nervous Diseases. With Confederation came increased money and this opened the door for greater numbers of nurses to pursue continuing education. Sixteen of the respondents availed of this educational opportunity. King, "I worked for a little while at the General…I was on the fourth floor where we had the psychiatric patients and Dr. O'Brien would visit daily. He asked me when we joined Confederation, if I would like to go to the university and study psychiatry. I was very honored by that and was pleased to be asked. In 1949 I went to McGill University and others went to Toronto. But I went alone to McGill and I was there for one year." Dewling, "We graduated in 1948 and in 1949 we were into Confederation and there were some monies around. Actually if you look at it, Government was always interested in educating nurses and there were always things that government was doing. The Minister of Health at the time, Dr. Miller had come to the General and...chosen four or five people from different areas...to go to the University of Toronto and come back and do some teaching. I went and spent twelve months there and came back to the General...it was amazing the things that we learned."

Doctor-Nurse Relationship: While many of the previously discussed external influences might be considered outside the control of nurses, it was the 'other' influences within their work world that created some of the respondents' most interesting stories. Throughout history, the doctor-nurse relationship has always been a topic for discussion. These women worked in an era when the only health care providers were either doctors or nurses. In a health care facility such as a hospital or a key health care service such as public health often the doctor was the one in charge whereas the nurse was the one who did the majority of patient care. These nurses' stories give some idea as to their workload and responsibility, the autonomy they had to assume in their practice, the power struggles they encountered and the nurses' resilience when challenged.

To appreciate their stories it is important to put their situations in context. In the 1930s prior to the establishment of the Cottage Hospital system very few doctors practiced outside of the larger urban centers in the province and then only those rural areas with a cottage hospital had direct access to a doctor. During World War II, the number of doctors in the system was reduced as many went to war. When doctors eventually began to work in the smaller communities, they were primarily salaried doctors, paid by Government, so their salary was not dependent on the number of patients they saw. Many of these nurses were used to working independently with significant responsibility and accountability in their practice settings. It is not surprising that as doctors increased in number within the system issues began to surface around each others' roles and responsibilities.

For the nurse working in rural areas of the province, she was it; she rarely had access to a physician if at all. She had to rely solely on her own knowledge and skills and did not always have the luxury of consulting with another health care provider. For the nurse in the hospital setting, things were somewhat different in that they had access to a doctor and resources although many times this was in selective circumstances. Tobin gives a sense of the level of independence and responsibility that a nurse had in a hospital setting. "[From 1944 to 1957] the nurses made a fair amount of decisions. The doctors did not live in. I think we only had one live in during the war. You had to be very careful [if you called him]. If they thought it was not necessary they would not come but they would tell you what to do. If there was anything that you were concerned about, you would tell them and they would make the decision whether or not to come. We had very little to do with doctors unless it was a new admission or an emergency." Even when Tobin returned as a night supervisor in the early 1960s, nurses still had a high level of independence and responsibility in their practice setting: "You made a lot of decisions on your own because there was only about four or five doctors. They would make their rounds between 7:00 and 8:00 o'clock in the night. The doctors were never called unless it was an emergency. We had no [house staff]. The night supervisors would make a lot of decisions. The student would notify us, they did not call the doctor on their own. We would make the decision if the doctor had to be called."

Many of the participants told stories of conflict between nurse and doctor as to who made decisions about nursing and patient care. Strong, "Before Dr. Roberts came [back from the war] I started classes. I thought that everyone should have the right attitude about the mentally ill. When Dr. Roberts came he was annoyed but I did not think I was doing anything wrong." Barrett, "I went in as Director of Nursing and they had a new administrator...from England. And we got along well. When he knew...the type of person I was. Because he called one of the head nurses down to his office one day and I didn't know anything about it. So anyway I went into him and I told him...I don't know what he said to me now...I can't remember...something about nursing. And I said, 'Are you telling me or asking me?' He said, 'No, Miss Wiley, I'm telling you.' And I said, 'Well don't you bother!' He never did it after. And...I must say, we got along. When he got oriented, you know, he was a pretty good administrator. After that, I had a free hand. And I remember one day...Dr. Baird...he did the first open-heart surgery. He was the first surgeon in Newfoundland to operate on the heart. And he came down to me this day – and they weren't doing what he wanted...Morphine...q4h [every four hours as necessary] he wanted. I said, 'Dr. Baird, how have you got the order written?' And he couldn't remember. So I said, 'Well let's go up and see.' So we went up and saw and he had it written q4h prn. 'Now,' I said, 'Dr. Baird, take off the prn (as necessary) and the nurses will give it every four hours.' But he was blaming the nurses. It went to the Head Nurse but, I mean, she was doing the right thing...and he couldn't get any satisfaction...so he moved up to me."

Tobin, "I can tell you of an incident when we were going to start a course for nursing assistants. Because they were just coming in off the street the same as the orderlies were. They were being paid the same at that time as a registered nurse. Anyway, we had this doctor who was Chief of Surgery and he came to me and told me that he would fire me if I went ahead with the course for nursing assistants. So, I told him to go ahead because I did not want the job anyway. At that time, I was Acting Director and really did not want the job. But I told him that we were going to have to start the course, which we did, and I did not get fired. [When the new Director came] there were altercations, but once the Medical Director realized...that she was the Nursing Director, everything ran smoothly."

Dewling, "We used to have this regulation in the General Hospital where, the doctors came in, made rounds with the nurse, gave the nurse verbal orders, and she wrote them in a book as she walked around and then transferred them to the individual charts afterwards. Anyway, one day I was with this particular patient on the surgical unit with a student and the doctor came, looked at the patient drinking a cup of tea. He had given the orders for her to drink liquids but she was not allowed to have milk and there was milk in the tea. Well, he let out one vicious scream to find out who put milk in the tea. At this point, the student was all colors. So, I said, 'I did.' I went back and I told him, 'You left an order for fluids and that is a fluid. If you wanted clear fluids, you should have left an order for clear fluids.' Then...I told the doctor I would see him in my office. Later, he came into my office all sweet and I told him not to dare do that to me. He knew that I was mad. I told him that I was here to teach nursing and I could not have doctors coming in making an ass out of me and of them. I also told him that he was very rude and I would not tolerate it. I then told him that I would not provide nursing for any of his patients unless he writes and signs every order. The next thing, I get a call from the Medical Superintendent. I went down and he told me that he had a complaint about my nursing and I told him my story. He told me that I was right and he did not want to get in the middle of it. That doctor did not speak to me for weeks. Well, right after that, there was a memo that came out stating that doctors had to write all orders and sign them."

What the nurse saw as providing comfort for her patients, the doctor sometimes saw as increasing their expectations as to the level of service they would receive. Griffen, "When I was here, (Gander) they used to come by the weigh freight...'cause there were no roads. And the first day I was there, in the night, they came...oh about twenty of them I suppose...from Gambo to Gander, to see the doctor. So I went down and I said, 'What are you doing?' They said, 'We want to see...are going to see the doctor.' And I said, 'Yeah, but he's not going to be in 'til 9:00 o'clock [the next morning].' Oh, they knew that. I mean, that wasn't their first visit. So I took pity on 'em and I started bringing them blankets and giving them hot chocolate and I had to call Dr. Paton in for a delivery. He said, 'Cleary, what are you doing?' And I said, 'These poor people down there, Dr. Paton,' I said, 'You got to give them blankets and pillows.' He said, 'Don't go past this door!' (which was the hospital part). He said, 'If they...if somebody dies, they'll come up and tell you.' He said, 'Tomorrow night, we'll have twice as many. Now look at the service you get in Gander now and they'll be back.' He said, 'Don't go past the door, for God's sake!' There were a couple of hotels in those days but I suppose they couldn't afford it. It was just a routine thing; they came up and sat in the waiting rooms 'til...the next morning."

When she worked at the Gander Airport, Griffen was also on duty the night one of the first jets landed in Gander. She wasn't above breaking the rules if she felt it was in the best interests of the people involved. Apparently while flying over the Atlantic, the plane lost altitude to the point that when it landed you could see the spray from the Atlantic covering the plane. When she went on board, the life rafts were in the plane. When she requested to see his vaccination certificate one of the passengers responded, "'You didn't appear over the Atlantic when we almost drowned, did you?' And I went up to somebody else and finally I came off because I had to call Dr. W. and I said 'Look there's panic going to be here...do I have to.' 'Yes, you have to check it [the plane]. We can't change the rules.' I said to Mr. Gettle, who was in charge of...who serviced the planes...'Let them off, will you? And he said 'Are you going to check them inside?' And I said 'I can't control them on the plane. I can't check them.' And he said 'Thank God! Somebody in National Health got sense.' And I said 'Well I hope you're behind me when I'm fired. Because I'm sure I'm going to be fired after this one (laughter).' You know, breaking the rules. I mean...they nearly mobbed the pilot; they had to take him outside. Apparently he had it on automatic pilot and he was in the plane...the outside, you know, in the passenger side when it started to go down."

However, not all nurses were prepared to take a stand against the doctor when it came to patient care issues. When Griffen worked in Corner Brook she encountered a patient care situation that caused her concern: "This one, R, was in charge and...one day I was there and I said, 'What's that one doing going down in the ward?' She said, 'Oh that's Doctor (I can't remember his name)'s secretary/nurse.' And I said, 'What's she doing in the ward?' She said, 'Oh she's doing a dressing.' And I said, 'What? She's doing a dressing?' She said, 'Yes, because the doctor doesn't like the person who's down there, the nurse that's down there.' So I said, 'Surely God he doesn't hate all of us? Sure you're worse than he is to let him do it!' That was the last straw! I mean, it's a wonder I wasn't fired. But she didn't fire me. I left before she fired me, I suppose."

In some cases, the encounters told of a time when the nurse had a broader role in the delivery of patient care services than today. On occasion there was some blurring of roles and responsibilities. If anything, the stories revealed the discrepancy between what the students learned in nursing school and what was expected of them in practice. Penney, "We spent two months in the case room alone so you were fairly learned [in Obstetrics]. You didn't call the doctor, I mean, because they didn't appreciate your calling if the lady wasn't ready, as they say. There were some of the doctors almost wanted [the baby] to come out and [say] 'Good morning,' you know (laughing), before...you called them. So they had to be pretty ready before you called them...one [doctor] was with Community Health. We always had one or two at Community Health and that's all they did. And we could call them. They did the clinics, and we could call them day or night. But you only called them if you really needed them. I mean, they didn't appreciate (laughing) being called out...you know, if it was a normal delivery."

While on duty one night at the Gander airport, Griffen found herself in trouble with the doctor: "Well it was a cargo flight and...the captain had to sign there was no sickness other than air sickness. So anyhow I heard the stewardess say to a crew member, 'What are they going to do with you?' And he said, 'Well they're going to keep me off 'til the next flight.' So I figured he was drunk. That's why I didn't tell Dr. W about my diagnosis. So anyhow I said to the captain, 'Are you sure there's nobody sick on this plane?' 'No, no,' he said, 'It's just a problem we have.' Anyhow, the man stayed off and the captain was just about to leave...when Dr. W called me and said, 'We have a west bound flight tonight.' And I said, 'Yes.' 'Anybody sick on it?' I said, 'No sir! There's nobody sick on it.' He said, 'Well do you know where I'm calling you from?' I said, 'I hope it's home.' He said, 'It's not. It's the hospital.' And he said he has some (I don't know if it was Measles) and 'You hold the flight.' And I said, 'Okay, I'll call Tower and tell them about the flight and I'll be up.' So when the Customs said to me, 'You know, you're gonna be killed.' I was only here not too long. I called Dr. Paton, and I said, 'Dr. Paton, how would I know?' He said, 'You wouldn't know.' (Measles usually come out on your chest first.) He said, 'You'd have to strip him. You'd think it was the flu, Cleary, don't worry about it.' So I figure now the best thing for me to do is get ahead of all this. So I went out in the main terminal and, when Dr. W arrived, he said 'Have you got the captain?' I said, 'Yes, he's waiting to see you.' And I said, 'But now I'd like to speak to you first, Dr. W.' He said, 'What's that?' And I said, 'Well don't yell at me because I can't stand being yelled at. If you're gonna fire me, fire me, but please don't yell at me.' And, my dear, we became the best of friends then because I was the right one for him!"

Some doctors just enjoyed using the power their position gave them. Dalley, "...but he [Dr. O]...always, sort of like, he wanted his own way. He was the only one that read my orders to me, you know, what to be doing. One of them was this one. I'll never forget. 'No patient to be allowed up on the ward without seeing the doctor.' Well this night I was on duty and this women came in...she was Dr. C's wife...but I didn't know her until she told me her name. And I said to the nurse's aide, 'Now you got to go over and call Dr. O...and tell him there's a patient here that got to be admitted. And when he came over and saw Mrs. C, I know he wasn't mad at me...because Mrs. C was one of his real good friends. He cursed on me, he swore on me, he did everything in the world. And I said to him, 'Dr. O, are you finished?' He looked up at me and said, 'Yes I think I am.' I said 'Dr. O, you were the very doctor that read the rules and regulations of this hospital to me. You told me I wasn't to allow anybody up on the ward without seeing a doctor' I said. 'Now the rule for one is the rule for all.' He never messed with me after that! When we were in the Operating Room he never called an instrument by name; he'd always point. And sometimes you'd pick up the wrong one; you wouldn't know which one he was pointing for. Oh! Wouldn't he curse!"

House, "Dr. O, he was...a good doctor and very strict...but still...he could be nice and I remember I was doing nights one night and I was sitting at the desk and he came up and he always wore sneakers and you wouldn't know he was near. And at the time we had a little boy with a temperature of 105°...so he came up to the desk and he said where was the little boy? And I told him what room he was in, so he went on. And instead of me jumping up to go with him, I finished what I was doing. So the next thing he came back and he said 'Who's more important around here? You or me?' And I said 'I think you are Dr. O.' 'Well,' he said 'Don't forget it.' And I was terrified! I thought, 'Oh my goodness!' So anyway he left and went downstairs again and the next thing, up he passed along...and he never said a word and opened the door to the women's ward and I jumped up and he said 'You remembered.' He went on again, you know. He was like that...but he was good...I know when I resigned, he tore up my resignation three times. So when I put in my resignation, he said 'Where are you going?' I said 'Corner Brook.' 'No, you're not!' He said (laughter). So anyway, finally I said, 'Well I'm going regardless'."

Some of the participants spoke quite highly of their doctor colleagues. Strong, "He [Dr. Grieves] had a great interest in it [psychiatry]...and he taught us a lot. He was the one who gave us our lectures and taught us about our own personality and viewing the patient as an individual and not putting them into a category [the notion of respect]. He made you think tenderly and we all loved him." Griffen spoke of the doctor's support of the nurses; "Dr. W...with National Health and Welfare...he was good to his staff; he did everything for us. We couldn't do anything wrong. He was fantastic with us, but...he was in charge. Dr. W was fantastic to his girls, as he called us. And, I mean, if somebody went in and said, 'Look, sure you can't sleep in that place,' he'd be up, my dear, fighting because his nurses couldn't sleep. He'd figured his nurses had to get the best. We were hated by some of 'em because of the best kind of attention."

In their working relationship, there was no doubt about the nurses' place in relation to the doctor or the pecking order. This is probably best reflected in Moakler's story of her time on the ship The *Lady Anderson*. "That was a great job...there was a staff on board – it was nine men and myself – and they treated me like a queen. The *Lady Anderson* was a beautiful looking ship; and there were two suites; the captain had one suite and the other suite was supposed to be for the doctor. So, of course, while I was on, I couldn't have a suite. I wasn't allowed to use the doctor's suite because I was a nurse even though we didn't have a doctor on board while I was there. But every now and then some doctor would come out from St. John's and stay on board and go along the coast and visit." Moakler had also experienced this attitude previously as a student, "I mean you never walked ahead of a doctor. You never walked in through a door, you always held the doors open for the doctor. You wouldn't get the nurses to do it now."

The era in which these women worked could be described as 'the best of times and the worst of times.' While they faced formidable challenges in their practices, they also revealed their strength, ingenuity and resilience in their response to them. They had a very clear sense of their role and responsibility as a nurse; it was to provide service to their patients and they did so without question. They were prepared to assert themselves but always did so in the interest of patient care and their profession.

PART 4 :
Then and Now

A question asked of the participants was how they thought nursing had changed or what they saw as the biggest changes over the course of their career in nursing. It elicited a myriad of responses as well as thoughts and feelings about their profession. This group of women had seen the explosion of technology in health care, the introduction of numerous groups of health care workers into the hospital setting, married women entering nursing school, men entering the nursing profession, the introduction of the nurses' union, their schools of nursing close, and nursing education move to the university, as well as a changing emphasis in nursing practice and health care delivery. But for many the most significant change was the loss of important symbols like their uniform and cap and what they thought this meant for nursing today. The comparisons between nursing in their day and today were inevitable. They talked of the changes they saw in nursing and health care and voiced their opinion of these changes. The feelings expressed about their own nursing career were probably the most enlightening and provided significant insight into who they were as nurses and women.

CHAPTER 10:
Changes in Nursing

"There was one thing that I didn't like, they took away our uniforms and caps. The caps were our dignity because we had to work for them." Merrigan (39)

Symbols and Traditions-Their Meaning: When talking about their time as student nurses, many of the respondents discussed the significance of their uniform and cap. For many of the participants, it was an important issue that nurses no longer wore a cap or a unique uniform. From their perspective, both had meaning not just to them but also within the system. Avery, "In the first year, you didn't get your cap until you passed your exams. At the Grace Hospital, for the first two years, we wore black stockings. Also, we wore plain royal blue uniforms under our bib and apron for the first three years. But our stockings changed and after six months we got stripes instead of just plain blue. So, you could tell by the uniform what year you were in. At the end of our second year, they decided that we could buy our rings and wear them to identify us as student nurses." Puddister, "The uniform when we first went in was blue stripes with a white background and a short apron...the first six months. Then we changed into a cap and bib with no apron. We wore that until we graduated. We then got the white dress and the black band on the hat. I believe all of that is gone out now." House, "And to see them, I mean, what they wear and oh...those uniforms...[and I mean the Grace hat was really distinctive]." Griffen, "We wore long sleeves, white...and they had great big cuffs on 'em. You'd be shot if you didn't have your cuffs on." Woodland, "[The cap signified] you had passed your exams...then you became a student nurse." Higgins, "You got your cap after six months, and we wore plain pink for the first year with your bib and apron. And then in the second and third year, you wore pink stripes."

Invisibility of Nursing: Some of the respondents' comments about the cap and uniform revealed what they saw as the impact for nursing in today's health care system: the invisibility of nursing. Giovannini, "I don't know if

I agree with doing away with the uniform. I found it difficult to recognize the RNs because there was only a name [tag]. I think if they had a white coat on or something like that it would be easier to distinguish them." Ashbourne, "They're up there like you or me with their street clothes on with no caps. So now Ross [her grandson in nursing] told me when I was down one day there awhile ago and he said that they were going to pin...apparently they give the student nurses...a pin instead of a cap because there were male nurses now." Sister Fabian, "I think the uniform has taken away something; you go on the floor now and you don't know who is who. I think if they had something unique it would help, because they are all dressed alike; the nurses, the laundry people, and the house-keeping staff. I was at the hospital a couple of years ago with my sister and I asked this worker if there was a nurse around and she told me that she was a nurse. She was a graduate and I felt so bad about not knowing it but there was no way for me to know that she was a nurse." Avery, "As a matter of fact, I don't see the nurses around as much now. I always felt that a nurse was somewhere around to be seen in my day. They were always in the schools and in the homes with three or four of them around in the district. I don't think they wear uniforms now either; we used to stick out like a sore thumb. I preferred my time to now. [You were distinctive.] But not only that, I always felt because we had uniforms, we always looked clean. Everyone else might still look clean, but back then you always looked ready to do a dressing." Higgins, "I see the changes in nursing that...a lot of the discipline, too much of it has gone and I don't like that. A lot of the professionalism has gone out of nursing. And I don't know... lately I've been trying to think about it. Is it since we joined the union? Although the union has been good, salary wise, I think the union has been good to get nurses their due, when the ARNN didn't seem to be strong enough to speak up. But whether as a union that's been too strong, I don't know. But to my mind, a lot of the professionalism is gone in everything. In the way they respond to the doctors by their first names. I knew a lot living in St. John's, but you'd never...it was always 'Doctor so-and-so' in front of the patient. You were staff, or whatever. If it was privately, you could/may speak different. Also in their dress. I don't mind not wearing their caps. When it goes for one to do without the caps, I don't mind that, but the whole dress system...I thought the biggest change was when ARNN wasn't the sole governing body...it has gone downhill ever since. I think to us ARNN wasn't that strong...but they were good. If you could only retain the goods things because...it got to do away with discipline. It has to be a balance or things get worse." Dalley probably best reflects how the changes impact on some of these older graduates: "We had to work hard and long hours but we enjoyed it. Health care is gone up in this hospital, they tell me...some only work eight hours now. And now they go on with not a cap on...you don't know them from the maid now. I went to visit somebody [in hospital]...and there was this girl standing up; she had on a red top and red slacks and I thought she was a visitor to the next bed...and Doug was there and he had...apparatus going into him, tubes and stuff...and something happened to it and she was fooling around with it, this girl was. And my dear, the sweat started to come out on me. Oh my Lord, I said! I was a nurse and I wouldn't know no more how to touch that than a fly. So finally his son came in. I said 'Bert, come here...for God's sake 'cause I'm nearly dead.' He said 'What's wrong, Aunt Eleanor.' I said, 'Look at that woman fooling around with you father's apparatus.' He said 'That's a nurse.' I said 'Oh my God! I thought she was a visitor' [because they don't look a bit professional now]. It certainly is not like the good old days...and back then you knew if you were a nursing student...you knew if you were from a different hospital. It's gone from bad to worse."

Public Perception of Nurses and Respect: As they talked about the changes in nursing, it was clear that these women had enjoyed a great deal of respect and were held in high esteem within the community. Giovaninni, "They were very, very kind. The people were marvelous; I was always ready to go dancing and they found that out. So if they found out I was going to stay the night, they would arrange a dance. Before I left La Scie, they had a new wharf built in Tilt Cove and after they knew that I was leaving they were after me to stay the night. So I said yes and they had a dance for me on the new wharf as a special goodbye. They were marvelous; I was very happy." Barrett, "But, you know, Newfoundland graduates could take their place anywhere...even back then. Yes especially back then...I was respected...and the nurses were...[but] you go with the flow today...and you're one of the crowd. Now I was one of the crowd because I remember when we had the graduation...and I came in last...and this nurse said to me. 'Mrs. Barrett, you should go in first because you're the Director.' I said, 'Look I'm the Director whether I'm first or last'." Sister Fabian, "I think there was a lot of respect for nurses; a nurse was up high. Any nurse that graduated had a lot of respect and they do today as well." When asked if it was unusual in 1945 for a single woman, to go aboard a boat with nine men to travel around the coast, Moakler responded, "It was very unusual for my family to think that I was out there but it wasn't unusual for me. Some people thought that I was sort of a devil-may-care but I was a very goodie-goodie and...they treated me so well and not one of them ever...I mean we'd pull up probably into Grand Bank and they'd be having a dance, and we'd all go to the dance and we'd all come home. There was no such thing as one person, one on one. We were a group and they treated me so well...especially the cook and I treated him as my father." Avery, "Everyone knew who I was. The ones [people in the community] who are still around and know who I am still call me Nurse Avery. People these days are all known by their first names but Mrs. Avery was my first name." House, "Well, I'll tell you now, where I play cards night time and they're always on first name basis but there's three or four and they insist on calling me Mrs. House. And I say, 'Look my name is Mary.' And 'No, you're Mrs. House. I remember you on the floor.' And you know they can't get away from it [because you're a nurse]." Hutchings, "Every place you went you had somewhere to stay...[and you didn't pay for it]...but they looked at it all as a privilege to have the nurse or minister stay with them." However, some believed that nursing no longer enjoyed this level of respect within the community. Merrigan, "Well, it seems like there is no respect for the graduates now." Barrett, "I don't have very much to say about that! I think that's gone down the drain. I don't think there's that much respect left for nurses today. I don't know why. I mean, they lost their uniforms. So be it! They lost their cap. They lost their white stockings. And now jewelry!" Ashbourne, "[They had] more [respect in the community] than they have now. I don't know. I mean, it was stricter. You didn't go around and call. Now, you hear them calling out one to the other all over the hospital which was never allowed you know."

Changing Focus - The Patient: Other changes that they believed had occurred during their career included a change in the focus of nursing as well as in nursing practices and nursing education. Sister Fabian, "I really think that there is no comparison. There is a comparison as far as care, I suppose, and the concern and compassion for the patient. As far as the workday goes, our days were a lot heavier in terms of work hours and manual work. In those days you did not have time to talk to the patient; today there is a lot of emphasis put on the patient and you can learn a lot more about them and their illness. Then, all we had was work, work, work; we had so little help that we did not have time to get to know our patients as well as we would have liked to." Tobin, "At that time, I think there was more emphasis put on what the ward looked like and how the beds looked before the patient was comfortable. The casters on the beds had to be turned in and every red blanket had to be the same so it would look good when you looked up the ward. I don't even know if we asked if the patient was comfortable...I think there was more emphasis put on the patient when I left nursing compared to when I began my career." Avery, "We did a lot more bedside care in my time than now. You felt close to the patients but you had so many to take care of." Story, "In my day the bed was more important than who was in it. The patient is the most important person in the hospital and they never complained about what we did to them because we would bath them down in a tub and go through their heads."

Changing Practices: Those who graduated in the 1920s and 30s saw the biggest changes in the practice of nursing. The introduction of antibiotics, disposable items and new categories of health care workers altered the role and responsibilities of the nurse in health care delivery. Giovaninni, "During my training, nurses never even took blood pressure; that was the doctor's job. Also, we never did many dressings until we were seen as a nurse. It was very hard in those days. For instance, if a doctor ordered a patient grains of Morphine, you would have to put a tablet into the syringe, shake it up and syringe off what was not necessary. It was not like today where everything is pre-packaged, we never had it that easy. If we got a patient with Pneumonia, quite a number of the patients used to die; there were no antibiotics. Antibiotics did not come into Newfoundland until after I came over here. So, if you went to a patient with Pneumonia, the first thing you did was take their temperature. Then you had to wash them and you even had to wash their mouth back then. Then, depending on where the Pneumonia was, you had to put Linseed...they would not last, so then...you used to have to cut the bark, crush it, and spread it over the patient to keep the heat in." Whiteway, "We used to have to make all our own dressings and package them. So you didn't have very much time in between. Oh there was a big difference [after 25 years]...you didn't have to get any dressings ready...that was all on trays then. And when you had to give a needle everything was [in a package]. Not like when we had to give needles. I used to have to boil the needle first [and boil up the solution in some cases]. I didn't have to do any [housecleaning because there was housekeeping staff]...and IVs were different too...we used to have to put the bottles up on the pole...a pole that we had to bring around...and we had two hot water bottles on either side to keep it warm (laughter). There used to be poultices...that was what we would use. And then all they gave 25 years later was a pill. Strong, "We did the lockers and swept the wards because there was no housekeeping staff. I didn't feel like a nurse because I was not trained as a nurse but I am glad that I stuck with it because psychiatric nursing was my field. Now, there are patients put into boarding houses with people that do not understand them and that is a very big change. Some thought that drugs were a genius and to an extent they are because for a Schizophrenic to be able to control their disease is very important." Merrigan, "It is much easier [now] because they have equipment to do it. We had to carry our supplies. Now they got a cart that they can wheel. I don't think patients stay [in hospital] long enough. There is so much difference today, it is much more convenient today compared to what we had."

Those who graduated in the 1940s were also subject to change in their workplace and practice. Tobin, "If we ever had to use Morphine, we had to light the Bunsen burner and mix up the amount of solution that we needed and take the little tablet out of the Morphine [container]. We put it onto the spoon and then mixed it with the heat. These were the things that took time. Certainly, we did not give much Demerol, Codeine, or Morphine. We stuck with whatever could be given by pill. I don't think it was too much different than what it is now. It was not as stressful, I would think, as it is today. It was routine patient care. When the sulfur drugs came in during 1943, they were considered the miracle workers. Then, we did not get Penicillin and Streptomycin until late 1944 or 1945." Nurse, "I think the biggest difference was...we had antibiotics so there was no...terribly long irrigations. And we had disposable things. Oh my heavens! Died and going to heaven (laughter)! The Bunsen burner and the little spoon so you put your pill in it and you had to waste...if you wanted to give a quarter of a grain, of something, you squirted off the other three parts, you know? Well, if I can put it right to the last part of it, I think there was too much emphasis...doing up charts. I know you've got to chart because you got to have your...it's legal, you've got to have it. I realize that. But it shouldn't...I don't know...it could be where I was from the old school. I mean, I always charted everything." Penney, "We didn't have any nursing assistants those days. We were it, you know!" House, "I suppose there wasn't that much difference not then but well, for instance, we didn't have to boil our needles when we'd give an injection. We had to boil our needles you know? They were disposable [when I came back]." Griffen, "Like now, if you spit up, they got a cleaner to come in and clean it up...at that time, you... cleaned the floors." Hutchings, "I had buckets for bringing in water from the well. The medications we had were very, very few. Compared to what they have today. I couldn't believe it when I went back in 1963 to see the pharmacology book." Higgins, "But still going back further when we trained and first graduated we did a lot of things that later on had to be done by medical students (laughter). In terms of things we were allowed to do [the role of the nurse lessened]...as time went on and when I was still in nursing that [a dressing] was done by medical students." Barron, "One of the big things, I don't know how people would handle it today...but then the way we worked! But you know about all the hours we worked. We sharpened our needles, we would patch the gloves, we would make the sponges, you know all the things to save money."

Changing Education: These women entered nursing at a time when they could walk in off the street, express an interest in nursing and if they met the requirements were accepted immediately into the program and began to work in the hospital. They learned primarily on the job so it is not surprising that some of them had difficulty with nursing education today. French, "The only thing I think about nursing these days is the training. In the training school you had to come in contact with the patients rather than theory. When you come to stick a needle into a patient it is not like sticking it into an orange...I am glad I trained in a hospital. Because I felt and still feel if you are in contact with the patients you are better off. You can have all of the theory you like but you do have to have contact. Approaching a book and approaching a person is different." Moakler, "In the last couple of years that I was working, they kept talking about the... nurse practitioner. And I kept thinking about, okay the wheel has already been invented. Why are they trying to invent this wheel? Because this is what we were doing for years. And now they're trying to start something new. To me it wasn't, but the last going off, I found that, in my opinion, they weren't turning out the calibre of nurses that we were. I really thought that we got terrific training and...I felt university girls got the education but we got the training...the practical experience." Barron, "The change in nursing education...has changed drastically. I know that it is wonderful to have a Masters degree in nursing and that you have got to have one to instruct, but I don't think a Bachelors degree or a Masters degree is the big qualification for an instructor. I think you need...it is wonderful to have that but you also need the practical experience and the experience under her belt...I think it [should be] two or three years as a nurse by the bedside in the clinical area and then go into teach. Then I think she will be better equipped, is probably the word, to teach nursing.

But I don't think (and I've seen this happen) coming right as a young girl into a BN program, then coming out of it and coming straight back...without even an RN exam passed and being put into a teaching position. I don't think they are able to teach the student what the student needs. I think you need that [the practical experience]. I'm not against the education part, I think that's wonderful to be able to book learn but I think the practical...I think the person doing this teaching has to be somebody who already has this experience and I think that's missing now."

For others, change in the way nurses were educated was vital and seen as positive. Nicholle, "They worked along with the Director of Nursing Services and ran the students...that was awful that was. If there wasn't any nurses on the floor they came over and took the students out of the classroom...and they put them on night duty. So when the nurse intern courses came in they took the nurse interns and put them on the floor, took full charge of them and we had the second and first years so that was the independence we had. We didn't have a soul in the school with degrees then...I was trying to make the school separate from nursing service. [Recently] I was up there [the hospital]...I saw more university graduates and students than I did our own...and they were ladies, they were smart, they knew what they were doing, they were mature and I could trust them. They're smart girls. I don't know how much experience some of them had but they were firm on their feet." Story, "It is very difficult to pin it [changes in nursing] down because I think it is an evolving thing and we were trying to make changes back then. I am not sure that we really succeeded at all. It is a gradual thing and everything is changing at the same time so it is hard to pinpoint any great moment. Perhaps the biggest thing was the introduction of the two plus one [nursing program]...where we would educate nurses and not train them. Because they would come out after six months with a cap and not know anything."

Thoughts and Feelings About Nursing: Probably the most surprising outcome to the question about changes was the respondents' expression of their feelings and thoughts about nursing. The majority positively commented about some aspect of their career and their profession and it was obvious that they loved what they did despite the hard work and difficult challenges. It would be easy to summarize the comments but only their own words can portray what being a nurse really meant to these women. Whiteway, "I came into training. I loved it! We used to have, you know, great times together. We were very close together." Williams, "Oh, they thought it [being a nurse] was just wonderful, you know? They thought there was nobody like me. It was a wonderful life, girl. I enjoyed it. I loved the water. I loved the boats. I loved it." French, "There was never a dull moment. It was good." Barrett, "I can truthfully say I had a wonderful career." Ashbourne, "I don't know [what I liked best] I liked it all (laughter). We enjoyed it, we had a good time...you worked what you had to do...so that's all you expected. You didn't look for anything else...there's too many Florence Nightingales now." Bruce, "I can very honestly say, that it [nursing] made me a finer person. I valued each year very much; it was a beautiful profession. I have probably mentioned it earlier in the conversation but it was a very happy time for me and it made me a finer person. I loved it. I'm so pleased to be back in touch. In particular in the museum where I see so many things that were in existence in my day, it is very rewarding. You can say I am a very happy older nurse." Nurse, "It's one thing that I didn't ever think of; I'm sure. I must have been alone on this, but I never once thought about making money in nursing, never thought of my future that I was going into something that I was going to make my life...make my living out of. That didn't occur to me...I think I was very immature...I think, not that it was service exactly but you did it to look forward to nursing. And it certainly...it was something that I was forever grateful that I had because, with a family...you know, not only financially but...it was just wonderful, just wonderful. It was certainly a wonderful experience...a real good career. I have no regrets about any of it except I would have taken it all a bit slower then. We were one big family because we were a small class." Avery, "Anyway it was a very rewarding and a really good career.. It was a great life and I felt when it was over I had a lot of things to think about...but nursing is very interesting." Penney, "You never knew when you went on in an evening, I mean just what you were going to be faced with before you came off. I enjoyed that; that was a challenge...enjoyed it very much...I enjoyed every aspect of it. I must say ...every aspect was interesting." Moakler, "I would like to be able to turn back time...we worked very hard in training, but looking back at it, we had a great time. And we learned a lot. They were very strict with us. I didn't think I was doing anything spectacular. Now it frightens me. When I think back....it wasn't unusual; it was expected of you. I felt I was helping somebody and that's what I went in training for...and people were so good to me...you appreciated it and they appreciated it." Nicholle, "I enjoyed every minute of it [being director of the school]...I had a good career." Taylor, "[It was a good life] very satisfying...it has changed...it's too technical. Not enough patient care. One doesn't know what to think; at least

I don't. [I would recommend nursing to people now] because there's a need for nurses. There's not very much encouragement to do nurse's training. They get into too much debt, I mean we didn't have to pay for our training. We paid a little bit. There's not much of an encouragement. They do go in but...go to the States because they can't pay off their debt. [For us] it wasn't only money. I mean this was a mission station at that point (Taylor went to Forteau as a missionary)." House, "Oh yes! [Nursing was a good choice]. When I go up now to visit, I think oh my, I wish I could go to work. It was fun though...even today I'd like to be back at it. When I worked on days, I didn't have as much contact with the patients....too much paper work...I enjoyed it though." King, "We just loved our nursing; it was our whole life. We were very happy together and by living together we got to know each other better. Next week, I am meeting my remaining classmates for lunch to celebrate it being 56 years since we entered training. Also, every June, both sections of the class [A and B] go to [a classmate's] and have a lobster dinner. We have not forgotten each other." Woodland, "Oh yes! I'd like to go back and do the whole thing over again. When I go visiting in hospital now and they call a 'nine' I want to jump and run. And when I first finished working and this would happen, I'd just automatically jump up. And I don't miss it until I get inside a hospital door. Oh I wouldn't nurse now if you paid me! I wouldn't want to go back now with the way things are with all the computers...and everything. We had patients come from the OR right straight to the floor. We didn't go to a special room or anything. Our suctions were not something you could plug into the wall...I would like bedside nursing now...I'd make a great nurses' aide...I like making people comfortable." Barron, "I really did love nursing that much...I don't know if I'm right or wrong but I know when I went into nursing it certainly wasn't for money, money was something...but as long as you had a bit to eat and didn't starve to death it didn't bother me. You know money wasn't the reason and I wonder now if a lot of people going into this profession are going in it for the career and the job; I don't know but I think unless they really and truly care and if they are not in it to help then they are in the wrong profession. And I think that is why there is discontent because you know we worked. I don't think physical work is going to kill you but you can't always be complaining. It is a commitment. It has to come from the heart. It's one of the hardest things to give up." Roche, "Everybody knew everybody else. You would never hear a janitor say that the job he was asked to do was not in his contract. Whatever had to be done was done. It was more of a family atmosphere." Given these women's feelings about their profession, it is not surprising that a tradition of nursing existed in many of their families. Some of the respondents entered nursing because they had a nurse in the family who had influenced their decision but the majority of women in this project had sisters, daughters, nieces, granddaughters and even grandsons who followed them into the profession.

There is no doubt that many of their patients touched the lives of these nurses, as evident throughout their recollections of their time in nursing. While all patients are important there are always those who stand out more than others in that (for whatever reason) they made an impact. Woodland shared stories of patients she cared for as children but was still was able to recognize them years later as young adults. Her stories give some sense of how important the nurses' relationship was with her patients. Woodland worked nights at the Janeway: "Many a night I sat in a rocking chair...in fact I went to Zeller's restaurant a little while ago and this young girl came by and I looked at her...and finally I said, 'Were you ever a patient at the Janeway?' She said 'Yes, I was there a long time.' And I said 'Is your name Tina?' And she said 'Yes.' And I said 'My dear, I spent more time rocking you.' And she said 'Mom said somebody down there had me spoiled.' Another night I was working and a big tall doctor came in...and I looked at him...the dark eyes...and I said 'Are you from Grand Falls?' And he said 'Yes.' And I said 'Is your name..?' And he said 'Yes.' And I said 'My son, I was in the case room when you were born.' His mother was very, very ill after she had him and...in hospital a couple of months...and I looked after him. He was my boy!"

Throughout the interviews, the participants' pride in their profession and their work permeated the discussions. It is small wonder that they had difficulty accepting the changes they observed in their profession, particularly the loss of the uniform. It is not that the uniform made them nurses as much as it made them visible to the people who needed them. They saw it as their duty to be out there for their patients and in their eyes, the uniform facilitated that. They perceived a connection between the loss of the uniform and a loss of respect for nursing.

While they acknowledged the value of many of the changes in their profession, particularly those that eased the nurses' workload, they grappled with others such as the changes in nursing education. For so many of these nurses the focus of their work had been their patients' comfort and well being and yet, increased patient focus was one of the positive changes in nursing that many of them identified. However, it was the fond memories of their time in nursing and their obvious joy when sharing them that best illustrated the importance of nursing in their lives. Their recollections told so much about what they had given to their patients and their profession and how they had shaped it for those of us who followed in their footsteps.

PARTICIPANTS NAMES
Schools of Nursing

When Graduated

1. Margaret (Dodd) Giovannini
   England, 1924

2. Ada (Gilliard) Oakley
   Grace Hospital, 1931

3. Edna (March) Whiteway
   General Hospital,1934

4. Ethel Williams
   Grace Hospital, 1935

5. Katherine (Fraser) Strong
   General Hospital, 1936

6. Phyllis Godden
   General Hospital, 1938

7. Jane (Lodge) Mifflin
   Grace Hospital, 1939

8. Eleanor (Jennings) Dalley
   Grace Hospital, 1939

9. Marcella (Woodrow) Merrigan
   Grace Hospital, 1939

10. Marcella French
    General Hospital, 1939

11. Phyllis (Wylie) Barrett
    General Hospital, 1941

12. Helen (Moore) Ashbourne
    General Hospital, 1942

13. Sr. Mary Fabian Hennebury

St. Clare's Hospital, 1942

14. Blanche (Williams) St. George
St. Clare's Hospital, 1942

15. Margot (Pike) Bruce
General Hospital, 1943

16. Mary (Hunt) Nurse
General Hospital, 1944

17. Gertrude (Farrell) Tobin
General Hospital, 1944

18. Mary (Cahill) Penney
St. Clare's Hospital, 1945

19. Elizabeth (Meadus) Avery
Grace Hospital, 1945

20. Lillian (Basha) Moakler
General Hospital, 1945

21. Margaret (Madden) Puddister
St. Clare's Hospital, 1947

22. Joan (Cleary) Griffen
St. Clare's Hospital, 1947

23. Rose Nicolle
General Hospital, 1947

24. Mary Taylor
England, 1947

25. Mary (Pynn) House
Grace Hospital, 1947

26. Joan (Evans) Higgins
General Hospital, 1948

27. Ruby (Skinner) Dewling
General Hospital, 1948

28. Janet Story
General Hospital, 1948

29. Ruth (Morgan) King

General Hospital, 1948

30. Jane (Clouston) Hutchings
    QE II – Montreal, 1948

31. Edith (Skinner) Woodland
    Grace Hospital, 1948

32. Mary (Morry) Barron
    St. Claire's Hospital, 1949

33. Kathleen Roche
    General Hospital, 1949